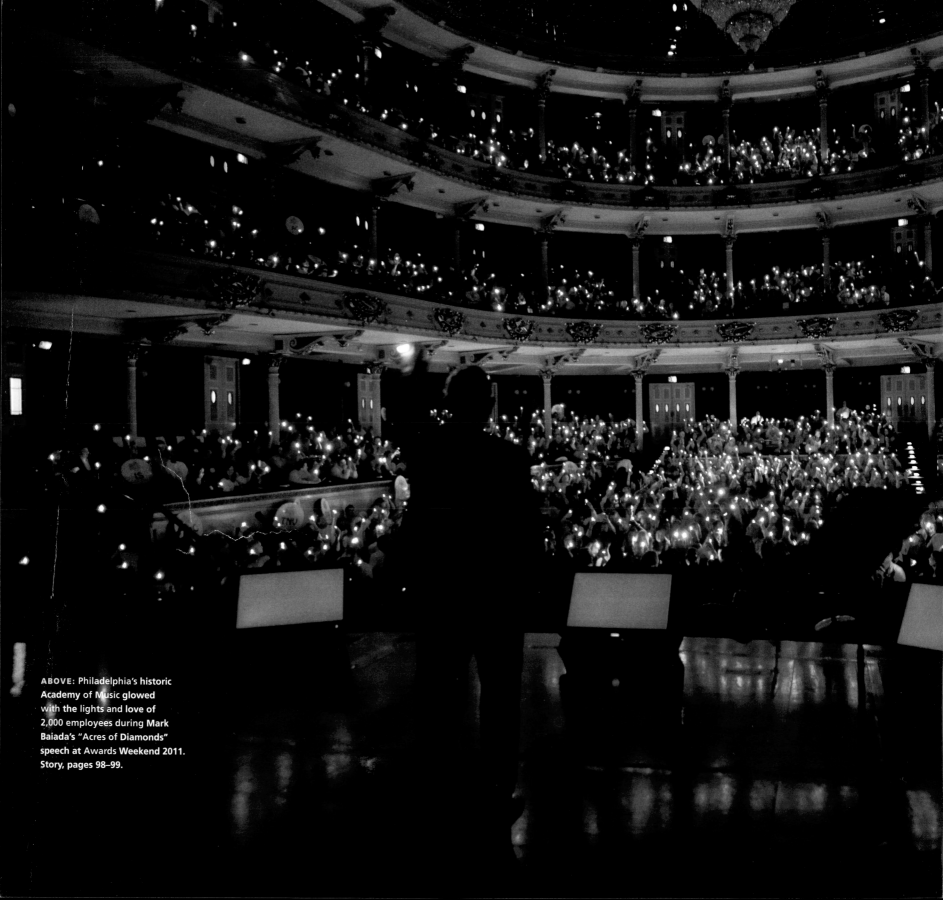

ABOVE: Philadelphia's historic Academy of Music glowed with the lights and love of 2,000 employees during Mark Baiada's "Acres of Diamonds" speech at Awards Weekend 2011. Story, pages 98–99.

BAYADA

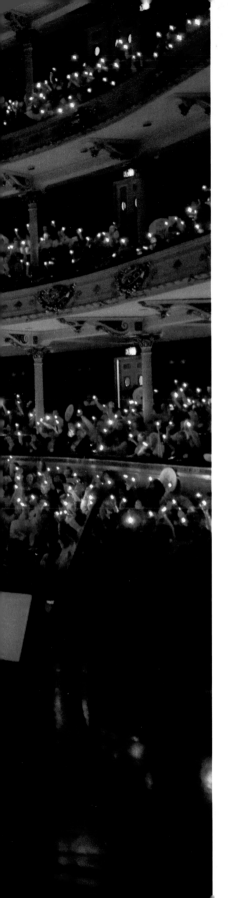

BAYADA

40 Years of Compassion, Excellence, and Reliability

BAYADA PRESS

BAYADA
40 Years of Compassion, Excellence, and Reliability

© 2015 BAYADA Home Health Care, Inc. All rights reserved.

ISBN: 978–0–9906012–2–7

Produced for BAYADA Press by CorporateHistory.net, Hasbrouck Heights, NJ

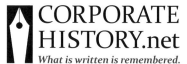

www.corporatehistory.net

AUTHOR: Christine McLaughlin

PROJECT MANAGER AND EDITOR: Marian Calabro

ART DIRECTOR AND PRODUCTION MANAGER: Christine Reynolds, Reynolds Design & Management, Waltham, MA

Printed by Penmor Lithographers, Lewiston, ME, using Creator Silk Text, Forest Stewardship Council Mixed Sources Certified Paper

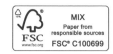

PHOTOGRAPHY CREDITS: The company expresses sincere thanks to clients, employees, and retirees for the use of their images, and to Chris Medlar for his photographic services. All images and artifacts appear courtesy of BAYADA Home Health Care and the Baiada family, except those listed below.

Page 13 (tie): Shutterstock. Page 16 (chicken) and page 22 (roll of quarters): iStockPhotos by Getty Images. Page 22 (Qwip® ad): Vintage Paper Ads.

CONTENTS

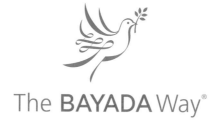

The BAYADA Way®

Our Mission

BAYADA Home Health Care has a special purpose — to help people have a safe home life with comfort, independence, and dignity. BAYADA Home Health Care provides nursing, rehabilitative, therapeutic, hospice, and assistive care services to children, adults, and seniors worldwide. We care for our clients 24 hours a day, 7 days a week.

Families coping with significant illness or disability need help and support while caring for a family member. Our goal at BAYADA is to provide the highest quality home health care services available. We believe our clients and their families deserve home health care delivered with **compassion, excellence,** *and* **reliability,** our BAYADA core values.

Our Vision

With a strong commitment from each of us, BAYADA will make it possible for millions of people worldwide to experience a better quality of life in the comfort of their own homes. We want to build and maintain a lasting legacy as the world's most compassionate and trusted team of home health care professionals. *We will accomplish our mission and achieve our vision by following our core beliefs and values.*

Our Beliefs

- We believe our clients come first.
- We believe our employees are our greatest asset.
- We believe that building relationships and working together are critical to our success as a community of compassionate caregivers.

- We believe we must demonstrate honesty and integrity at all times.
- We believe in providing community service where we live and work.
- We believe it is our responsibility to strengthen the organization's financial foundation and to support its growth.

Our Values

Our work is guided by our fundamental values.

Compassion—Our clients and their families feel cared for and supported.

Excellence—We provide home health care services to our clients with the highest professional, ethical, and safety standards.

Reliability—Our clients and their families can rely on us and are able to live their lives to the fullest, with a sense of well-being, dignity, and trust.

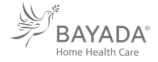

BAYADA®
Home Health Care

Compassion. Excellence. Reliability.

INTRODUCTION

It's hard to believe that BAYADA Home Health Care has come so far since 1975, when I began the company from a single office in Philadelphia. Those early years set the course for where we are now. Today, nearly 3,000 office employees help make it possible for more than 20,000 field employees from 290 offices in 21 states and India to serve more than 26,000 clients a week.

However, numbers aren't the true measure of success. It's the relief a mother feels, knowing she can sleep peacefully at night while her medically fragile child is under the skillful, watchful eye of her BAYADA Nurse. It's the senior citizen who can remain living independently at home with the helping hand of his BAYADA Home Health Aide. It's the home health aide who says, "I love my job. I wouldn't want to work anywhere else."

When I reflect on these past 40 years, these are the things that define success to me. You can't assign a value to the priceless feeling of being in the comfort of home. Or knowing that because of the work you do every day, more people can stay in their homes with their loved ones and treasured memories.

I continue to be humbled by the trust our clients place in us every time one of our caregivers enters their home, and I feel good knowing that BAYADA has made a real difference in the lives of our clients. Our clients have made a difference in our lives, as well, inspiring us every day to work hard to provide the very best home health care services. They deserve no less.

Although we continue to grow and serve more people each year, we never lose sight of our original mission of helping every client have a safe home life with comfort, independence, and dignity. Helping people has been—and will always be—our singular purpose. It is the driving force behind *The BAYADA Way,* our company philosophy, and the heart of everything we do.

I remain grateful to our BAYADA employees for the care they provide and the love they show to our clients. Our employees are truly the heart of home care, and paramount to BAYADA's success, helping us to help more people each year.

We may be a big company now, but we are a big company with an even bigger heart. And regardless of the roles we all play, we are really just people helping people live better lives—with compassion, excellence, and reliability.

As a reflection of BAYADA over the past 40 years, I hope that this book will commemorate our beginnings, our growth, and our accomplishments, and, perhaps, most significantly, capture the everlasting spirit of *The BAYADA Way.*

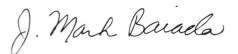

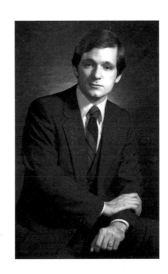

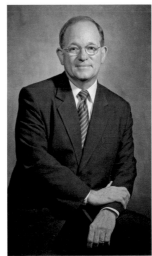

CHAPTER ONE

The Early Years
"A Community of Compassionate Caregivers"

BELOW AND RIGHT:
Mark Baiada has thought hard about goals from the very start. He wrote the chart and the lists below when the company was eight months old.

---

5 year Plan   RN Home Care   8-19-79

1. 20 Offices - company owned
2. 5% EBT   20% Return on Equity   on Pmt.
3. Capital - Internal
   - maybe some debt for A/R
4. Personnel
   - Goal oriented
   - Promotable Mgmt. Group
   - Hard workers
   - Smart
5. Finance - central control of payroll & billing
   - central control of purchasing & payables
   - Cent. Cntrol control of budgets
   - Weekly, Monthly, Quarterly, Annual
6. Obstacles - Principle of Standardization
7. Obstacles (1) Marketing
   (2) People Personnel
   (3) Recruiting
   (4) Field Staff Mgmt. (Who is available?)
   (5) Performance Evaluation - Testing
   (6) Training

Objective -
1. Long range - Build a large organization, with good profit
2. Short range - Get Phila. running real smoothly so it's a model for other areas. Goal for Jan. 1 is $7,000 week, large staff, positive cash flow, good payroll, billing, and accounting system, formal pay schedules, Expansion plan, more free time for me, good office personnel

Strategy
1. recruit
2. Hire a bookeeper/sec., then get fin. statements to see if we can hire another service coordinator
3. Free my time for mgmt.
4. Get financial statements and projections.
5. Stick to the plan

Model Organization Plan

```
                    Director
                       |
      _____|_____
     |            |            |                |
  Service      Nursing Dir   Bookeeper          |
  Coordinator                                    |
     |                                           |
  Service Coor.                                Clerk
```

> *"I like people and see the best in them."*
> J. MARK BAIADA

BELOW: Mark's love of parties and celebrations began in his childhood home.

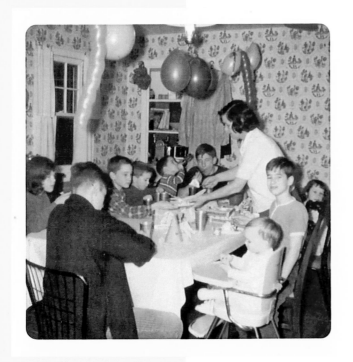

The history of BAYADA Home Health Care begins with the history of its founder, Joseph Mark Baiada. The son of an Italian father and immigrant Serbian mother, and the eldest of six brothers, Mark grew up in a close-knit family who shared a solid foundation of caring, love, and respect for others.

Mark's parents, Laurence (Larry), a former Naval officer, and Anne, a former Navy WAVE, fostered a can-do attitude, independent thinking, and a strong work ethic in their six sons. They also cultivated the softer side, emphasizing the importance of humility, sensitivity, and loyalty to family. Discipline could be strict, but laughter also echoed through the family's big blue house in Delanco, New Jersey, a small town across the river from Philadelphia. Mark had the additional guidance of his tough yet lovable Italian grandmother, Caterina Baiada, who lived with the family. Like all the Baiadas, she had plenty of energy and a good sense of humor. An extended family of aunts, uncles, and cousins gathered regularly for holiday feasts and birthday parties, to celebrate the arrival of babies and to mourn the passing of loved ones as well.

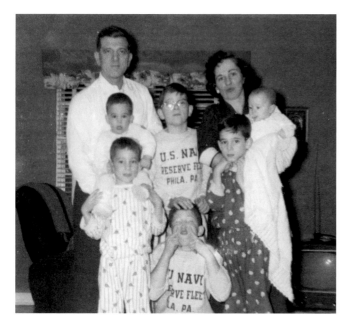

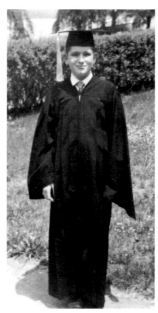

TOP ROW: The Baiada family with Mark, the oldest of the six sons, standing between his parents.

Mark at his eighth grade graduation. He is a graduate of Holy Cross High School in Delran, New Jersey.

BOTTOM ROW: Mark took seriously the Boy Scout values of trustworthiness and good citizenship.

Mark holding his brother Mel, circa 1959.

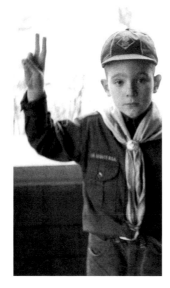

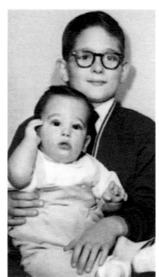

Mark took all of his early life lessons to heart. Asked to boil them down into two words, he doesn't hesitate: "Family first."

Surrounded by entrepreneurism through his parents' small insurance agency in rural Burlington County, New Jersey, as well as several of his relatives' small businesses, Mark absorbed their example. He knew from a young age that he wanted to own his own business, despite the long hours and hard work he witnessed daily.

"Work's no problem. I like to work," Mark says. While in Catholic school, he embraced the challenge of selling Christmas cards door to door. With a partner, he raised the most money for his school and earned the top prize.

While a solid work ethic was something he learned from his family, Mark's Catholic school education influenced him as well. Religion and values were very important to Mark. From a young age he even thought a lot about becoming a priest, until, as he says jokingly, "I discovered girls."

Hard work has always been part of being a Baiada. Mark and his brothers worked together to accomplish projects that often involved physical labor, developing close bonds and sharing laughs along the way. One of his grandmom's roles was to act as the taskmaster who kept the young workers on track. "We would egg her on and say that one of my brothers stopped working, even if he didn't. If anybody 'stopped,' she would be all over him," Mark remembers with a smile.

One family project had particular significance: In the early 1960s, Mark's parents decided that the family's home in Delanco needed a sea wall. It wasn't an idle notion, as the property bordered the Delaware River. Rather than hire a contractor, Larry assigned the job to his sons with one simple instruction: "Figure it out." Together, they did. The job took a full summer to complete—providing tangible evidence of the Baiada family virtues of patience, persistence, confidence, and thrift not for thrift's sake but in service of a bigger vision.

Although the family no longer owns that house, the sloping sea wall still stands. Mark's founding and nurturing of the company that would become BAYADA Home Health Care can be compared to the building of that wall. In fact, when asked how Mark's upbringing influenced his life and business, his son David has a one-sentence answer: "It's all about the sea wall story."

Certainly, the phrases "family first" and "figure it out" have echoed at BAYADA over the years. Just as the Baiadas encouraged a can-do attitude in their sons, Mark has built it into the structure and culture of the company.

Likewise, Mark's strong ties with his family have influenced his business in a profound way. He truly cared about making a difference for others, and he loved to help people. Mark's humility, his selfless frugality, and his sensitivity to others would serve as part of the architecture of his future company.

Deciding on home health care

Believing that a solid business degree would help him chart his entrepreneurial path, Mark dedicated himself to higher education. While commuting to Rutgers University in Camden, New Jersey, he also worked part-time at his

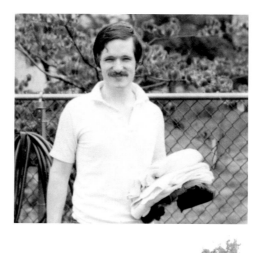

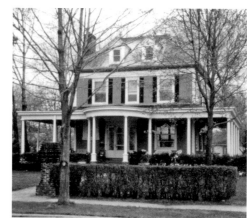

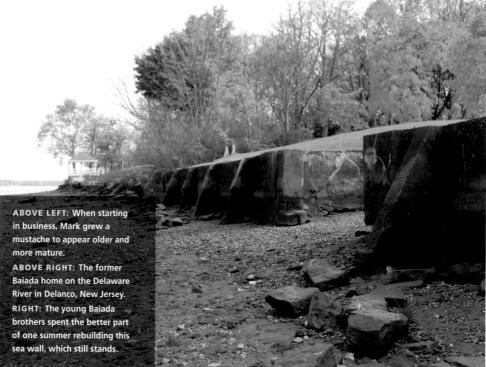

ABOVE LEFT: When starting in business, Mark grew a mustache to appear older and more mature.
ABOVE RIGHT: The former Baiada home on the Delaware River in Delanco, New Jersey.
RIGHT: The young Baiada brothers spent the better part of one summer rebuilding this sea wall, which still stands.

father's company, Baiada Insurance Agency. He finished at Rutgers in New Brunswick with a BA in 1969, becoming one of his family's first college graduates, and earned an MBA at Rutgers, Newark in 1970. After graduation, Mark worked as a market researcher at the American Thread Company in Stamford, Connecticut, and then at Avon Products in New York City. While he did very well, his corporate success was a means to an end—the goal of owning his own business. He voraciously read business books, articles, and annual reports. He admired the success and wisdom of Benjamin Franklin, Andrew Carnegie, and IBM founder Thomas Watson. To learn more about managing groups and activities, he led a Cub Scout pack. And on Wednesdays and Sundays, Mark

studied the business opportunities advertisements in *The New York Times* in search of a good fit.

He had clear criteria for the business selection. First, the business had to help people and make a difference in their lives. Second, it had to meet a growing need and be something to which he could devote his life's work. Third, it should be reproducible and expandable from coast to coast. Fourth and most immediately, he had to be able to start it on his savings of $16,000.

With these factors in mind, Mark decided to research one new business per month. First, he considered early child-hood education as a meaningful possibility. It had potential, especially because more mothers of young children were working outside the home. But Mark did not feel equipped to shape and mold young children's minds, as he did not have a background in education. Then, after seeing a bill-board for an auto painting chain seeking franchises, Mark briefly diverted from his criteria and explored that idea by repainting the beat-up old Volkswagen Bug at his parents' house. Curiously, he chose a shade much like today's "BAYADA red." However, he quickly realized that this would not be a fulfilling option.

Next, Mark thought about starting a nursing home. His father's cousin Josephine Healey—affectionately known as Little Jo—had previously worked at one, so he visited her to learn more about it. It was a fortuitous encounter, as she now happened to be working as a live-in home health aide for a local home health care agency. That kind of work interested him far more than nursing homes did. Perhaps it was because an image close to his heart—his

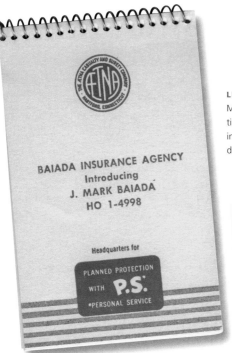

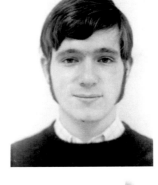

LEFT TO RIGHT: Mark worked part-time at the family insurance agency during college.

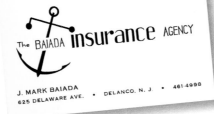

grandmom—tugged at him. She was getting older, although she was still quite independent. He knew that if she became sick or infirm, she could easily rely on family support. Many families weren't as lucky, he realized.

Some time later, Mark saw an ad for a local home health care company. Suddenly all of the pieces of the puzzle fell in place: "I saw the need, and I started to see a solution." With research, he determined that several agencies were finding success, and he thought, "I can do that." Mark further explored the market and liked what he found. The field was growing. A profession that involved intense human interaction, often in difficult circumstances, didn't faze him. "I like people and see the best in them. Not everybody does," he says with a smile.

Although most home health care agencies were still small and independent, a few regional and national chains had formed by the early 1970s. The biggest ones were spinoffs of staffing agencies that applied the "office temp" model to home care. In 1973, Mark answered an ad in *The Wall Street Journal* from one such agency that sold franchises. Its sales rep invited Mark and his wife at the time, Peggy Morrison, to meet him at the bar of the Roosevelt Hotel in midtown Manhattan. Upon shaking hands with them and taking a closer look, the man asked, "Are you old enough to drink?"

"It was really quite comical," says Peggy. "We did look like we were about 12 years old at the time."

In fact, Mark was 26. They listened politely to the sales pitch, and Mark asked plenty of questions. Seeking out information from colleagues and competitors is another

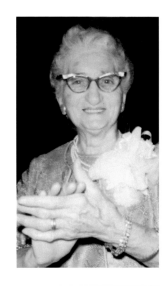

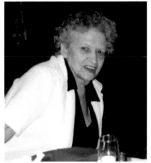

lifelong Baiada trait. True entrepreneurs—people who build real or metaphorical sea walls from scratch—are rarely content with franchises. Mark decided that he had enough background to start a business by himself and that he didn't need to pay franchise fees or be limited to a restricted geographic territory.

In 1974, the Baiadas moved to Philadelphia with a better understanding of the home health care industry. Why that city? Mark couldn't incubate an independent start-up in New York City on $16,000. He still loved Burlington County, but it was too sparsely populated. Philadelphia was "just right," with fairly low overhead costs and a population of 1.6 million. It also had a good public transport system, which would make staffing cases easier.

ABOVE AND LEFT: Two factors helped inspire Mark to create a home health care business: the aging of his grandmother, Caterina, and encouragement from his father's cousin "Little Jo," who worked as a home health aide.

BELOW: Mark likes professionals to look professional. That's why male office employees still wear ties to work.

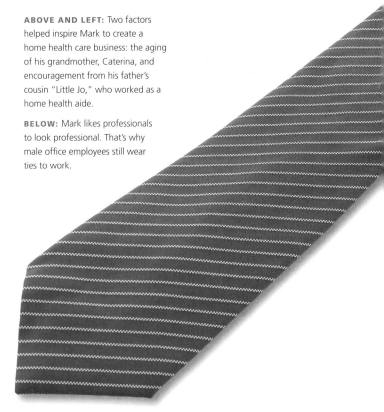

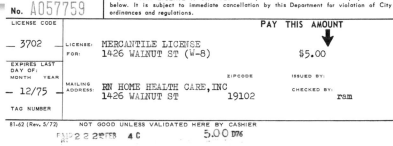

RESUME

Martha Jane Bodor
2701 East Orvilla Road
Hatfield, Pennsylvania 19440
215-822-9516

1/11 interview
for a, wellspoken, intelligent
but green

Green suit
maroon coat
long tight + board
hair

PROFESSIONAL OBJECTIVE: Psychology, counseling, or social service occupations.

Interest areas:

1. Children: emotionally disturbed, learning disabled, mentally retarded, orphanage work

2. Adolescents: emotionally disturbed, drug counseling

3. Adults: emotionally disturbed, counseling, social services

4. Research work

EDUCATION: Muhlenberg College. Allentown, Pennsylvania. A.B. 1974. *Overall 2.8 (Maj) 3.0*

Double major in psychology and social science. 41 credit hours of psychology including experimental research, case studies, psychological testing and work with emotionally disturbed children, learning disabled children, mental retardates and mentally disturbed adults. 28 credit hours of social science (not including psychology), primarily involving sociology.

EXPERIENCE: *＊ Please refer to second page*

1972-1974　Fieldwork: Allentown State Hospital in the Special Education Department; some work experience with "Haven House" in Northampton County; experiences with Lehigh County classes for mentally and emotionally disturbed children and learning disabled children. (References available)

1971-1974　Muhlenberg College. Allentown, Pennsylvania. Served as aid in Registrar's office throughout college career (work-grant: approximately 15 hours per week). Responsible for all transcript requests and other office duties. (References available) *M. Roland Dedek* *Betty Miller 1-433-3191*

were's her back neat, tidy, clean. Punctual, conscientious, gets along with all, One of best ever had

1973　Partime temporary office help. Norristown, Pennsylvania. Receptionist and light secretarial duties.

1968-1973　Keyat

LICENSE

CITY OF PHILADELPHIA
DEPT. OF LICENSES AND INSPECTIONS

DISPLAY PROMINENTLY
If required by law.

THIS LICENSE IS GRANTED to the person and location and for the purpose stated below. It is subject to immediate cancellation by this Department for violation of City ordinances and regulations.

No. A057759

LICENSE CODE

＿ 3702　LICENSE: MERCANTILE LICENSE
　　　　　FOR: 1426 WALNUT ST (W-8)

PAY THIS AMOUNT　↓
$5.00

EXPIRES LAST DAY OF:
MONTH　YEAR

＿ 12/75 ＿

MAILING ADDRESS: RN HOME HEALTH CARE, INC
1426 WALNUT ST　19102

ZIPCODE

ISSUED BY:

CHECKED BY:
ram

TAG NUMBER

81-62 (Rev. 5/72)　NOT GOOD UNLESS VALIDATED HERE BY CASHIER
FEB 22 22 FEB　4 C　5.00 D76

ABOVE: Mark and Marty Bodor, the first employee he hired.

LEFT: Marty's resume with Mark's notes: "1/11 interview, well spoken, intelligent but green." On January 14, she sent a thank-you letter with the salutation "Dear Mr. Daiaga." Mark didn't hold the misspelling against her.

BELOW: The company's first city business license cost $5.

Laying the groundwork

Mark believed he had the formula for success. It seemed simple: You hire good home health aides who, of course, will be compassionate, reliable, and do an excellent job caring for the clients. You treat your employees like family, and they in turn treat clients like family. From there, you grow the business. He admits he was naïve. "Here I am, age 27. I've never hired anybody. I've never fired anybody. You assume, 'Everyone is like me,' especially people doing this kind of work." Mark may have been inexperienced, but he was mature in the way that mattered most: He emphasized the core values that would later be defined as *The BAYADA Way.*

As he soon discovered, however, establishing the business would involve flexibility and patience. Like most employers in pre-internet days, Mark turned to daily and weekly newspapers. To find clients, he placed ads under "Situations Wanted" in *The Philadelphia Inquirer* and later in *The Jewish Exponent.* To find office and field staff, he used the *Inquirer's* "Help Wanted" section.

One of the first office employee interviewees was Marty (Martha) Bodor (now Marty Boughey). Fresh out of college, Marty called the number in the ad and talked to Mark personally.

"He set up the interview. Mark did not yet have an office, so he proposed that I meet him in the lobby of the Jefferson Hospital Alumnae Hall. My dad just flipped out. He's thinking this is some kind of hoax or mass murderer or something," laughs Marty. "So he said, 'I'm going with you.'" Although she was embarrassed and tried to talk him out of it, Marty's dad prevailed. On a cold December day in 1974, they met Mark, who was clean-cut, dressed professionally in a suit, and was completely disarming. "Mark introduced himself. He's a friendly, nice guy, and my dad said, 'cool' and he turned around and walked out. For the rest of my dad's life, they were friends, and the three of us often had lunch together," says Marty.

Marty started in January as the company's first Client Services Manager (or Staff Supervisor at the time). Next, Mark hired Bev Altman, RN, a part-time employee who helped with marketing. While Mark devoted himself to the fledgling business, Peggy worked full-time at Jefferson Hospital as a social worker. "We started on a bare-bones budget," says Mark, adding he did everything himself, from incorporating the company to designing the first logo and the business forms to performing the payroll and accounting services.

Opening the doors

In January 1975, the newly incorporated RN Home Health Care opened for business in sublet space on the second floor of 1426 Walnut Street in Philadelphia. Mark, Marty, and Bev began to admit a handful of clients, mostly seniors needing home health aide services. The aides were hired based on experience, their interview, and references; they were also tested on their knowledge of the sprawling network of buses, streetcars, and trains run by the Southeastern Pennsylvania Transportation Authority, better known as SEPTA.

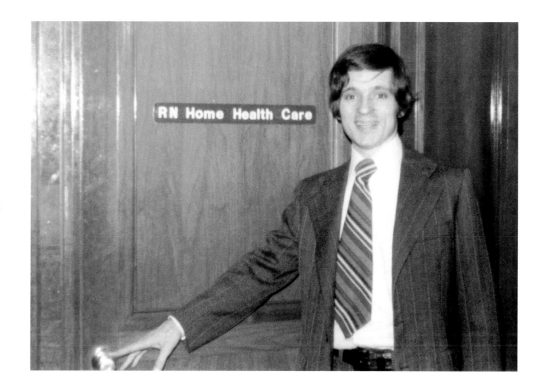

ABOVE: The enthusiastic founder at the door of the first office, located at 1426 Walnut Street, Philadelphia, Pennsylvania.

As the managers quickly learned, employees "called out" far more often than expected. In home health care parlance, a callout means that the field employee calls in sick or has another reason for not being able to go to a scheduled shift. Then as now, if there's a callout from a field employee, the manager in charge has to quickly figure out how to cover the shift.

"If there was a callout, you had to find the right person in a narrow window of time. We worked hard together, and felt fully accountable that we needed to figure it out. We

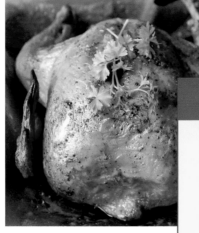

SEPTA strikes and the chicken callout story

Philadelphians of a certain age well remember the numerous SEPTA transportation strikes of the 1970s and 1980s, in which covering cases became a gigantic undertaking. BAYADA's supervisors and field employees went into "all hands on deck" mode. They began their workday several hours earlier than usual. Employees with cars volunteered as shuttle bugs to pick up and transport aides and nurses. Division Director Marion Fiero still laughs when she recalls the "chicken story," in which she diligently pursued a home health care aide named Marge to work as a live-in for a homebound client during the SEPTA strike. The dialogue proceeded like this:

Marge: Gosh, if you'd called me before I put my chicken in the oven, I would have said yes.

Marion: How long does it take to cook your chicken? We can cook your chicken there. I'll pick you up, you and the chicken.

Marge: No, no, no, it'll ruin the chicken.

Marion: Okay, well, how long will it take you to cook that chicken?

Marge: It'll be ready by seven o'clock.

Marion: I'll come at seven o'clock.

"I called her again from the office and I said 'Okay, I'm going to come now—is your chicken ready?'" Marion recalls. "My coworkers Marty Soroka and David Roarty went with me in my old jalopy. We picked up Marge and her chicken and her bag. She took care of that client until the client passed away." 🌿

RIGHT: Employees persevered through Philadelphia's disruptive transit strikes. "All hands on deck" has always been part of the company's work ethic. Featured in this 1981 company newsletter photo were Dana Axelrod, Carole McMahon, Marion Fiero, and Linda Siessel.

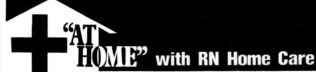

The Newsletter of RN Home Care   MARCH 1981

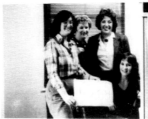

RN HOME CARE HANDLES SEPTA STRIKE.

"Shuttlebugs" Transport Aides

Some RN Home Care "Shuttlebugs."

Office and field supervisors organized to shuttle our Home Health Aides and Homemakers during the SEPTA strike to work. Our Aides are committed to providing care for our clients and where no other alternate transportation existed, our supervisors arranged car shuttles to make sure all our clients received continuous care.

In order to cover all our cases it was necessary for our supervisors and field employees to begin their work day several hours ahead of time. Our "Shuttlebugs" picked up our Aides at various locations in the City and shuttled them to their cases in Philadelphia and the surrounding suburbs.

Everyone has made an extra effort in working to overcome a difficult situation. This is a great example of how our team is committed to providing excellent services to all our clients.

George Knight Goes The Extra Miles

George Knight, an RN Home Care Attendent, travels two to three hours to go to his case during the strike. At dawn he walks 15 blocks from his East Germantown home to the train station. He travels to the next station and waits to transfer to another train bound for Norristown. Once in Norristown he walks blocks again to his client's home. At dusk he backtracks his way home.

George provides daily care to a young quadriplegic man. He promised his client he would not let him down during the strike. He is enroute for hours each day to keep his promise.

Director Thanks Staff

I want to thank all the RN Home Care employees for the extra effort in meeting our goal of continuous client service during the SEPTA strike. The cooperation displayed makes me proud.

The Field Staff was great: getting rides, walking (in some cases miles a day), taking on new cases, re-arranging schedules, working longer hours, or being shuttlebugs. The Office Staff did a fine job in planning and executing the Strike Plan. It took many hours of extra work, rearranging schedules many times over, making thousands of phone calls, and taking the responsibility for covering their cases properly.

On behalf of myself and our clients — *Thank You.*

J. Mark Baiada

knew what was expected and that we had to come through for the clients," says Linda Siessel, who joined the company in 1980 and is now Chief Operating Officer, Home Care Services, based in Morristown, New Jersey. "At the end of the day, it felt good to see the results and to hear the appreciation from clients."

Camaraderie developed fast in those years. There's something about the start-up phase of a business that turns colleagues into lifelong friends who become as close as family. Maybe it's the team-like environment, the shared challenge of operating on a shoestring budget, or the collective long hours. For these reasons and more, unshakable bonds are forged—as they certainly were during the early years of RN Home Health Care.

When another Marty came aboard—Marty (Martha) Soroka, who started in 1977—she was amazed that the founder and president's office consisted of a card table and a stool inside the utility closet. Mark had moved there temporarily to accommodate the growing staff.

The close-knit bunch worked long hours together, and Mark appreciated them. As a perk on hot summer days, he rented a room at the Holiday Inn next door so staff could go for swims. "During the day, we took turns going to the hotel pool and at the end of the day, we all went and had a little party," says Marty Soroka, Division Director of the Personal Care Assistant office in Philadelphia.

Laughs abounded, often to relieve stress but sometimes at Mark's expense. One day, he entered the office excited about his new "negative ion generator." He explained that

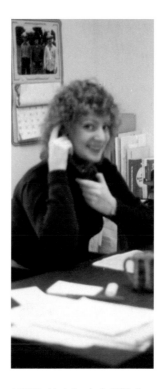

ABOVE: Marty Soroka in 1981. As a Service Coordinator (now Client Services Manager), Marty arranged homemaker service for elderly clients in north central Philadelphia.

it would eliminate negativity and make everyone happier. "Most of us were afraid of going near it because we thought we could get cancer from it," says Marty (Bodor) Boughey. "But Marty Soroka volunteered to put it on her desk. When we went to talk to her, we all would walk a big circle around her."

Landing the first major contract

The start-up phase involved a lot of prospecting. Mark tried to drum up referrals by calling local hospitals to let them know about his new agency. He continued placing ads in newspapers. "I was very research-oriented and would keep track of how many calls we received and how many turned to cases. I remember I wanted to get a new case a day," he says, adding that it took less than six months to meet his goal.

As the company started growing, so did the Baiada family. In 1976, Peggy was pregnant. While Mark and Peggy were busy preparing for their exciting new addition at home, Mark was also very busy at work. Mark and Marty (Bodor) Boughey were collaborating on an important proposal that could secure a contract with the Philadelphia Corporation for Aging™, which provided thousands of low-income senior citizens with home care services. Itself a nonprofit, at first PCA had hired only nonprofit agencies as providers. Some people in the industry exhibited a subtle bias against privately owned proprietary agencies like RN Home Health Care, despite the fact that profit margins were typically low. RN Home Health Care passed the first screening, and Mark was scheduled to meet with PCA officials on Wednesday, November 3, to bid for a major contract. It would be the biggest presentation of his life.

The night before the presentation, while ironing Mark's shirts and watching television coverage of the election of President Jimmy Carter, Peggy went into labor. Mark called Marty to let her know that she would have to handle the presentation. "I was in a panic. A dead panic," Marty remembers. "Then I thought, 'Well, I've got to go do this.' And somehow, I did it."

In fact, she won the contract for RN Home Health Care—a contract that is still active in BAYADA Home Health Care's fortieth year. Marty speculates on her success: "I think it was a combination of me being so young and scared, and the PCA people being so impressed that this young businessman, Mark, would fork over this opportunity and choose to be with his family." What's more, because the contract had to be rebid every year, Mark attended the 1977 meeting with a photo of his one-year-old son, David, to proudly show the committee.

Two landmarks

David Baiada was born the same day RN Home Health Care landed its first PCA contract, a landmark in the company's history. That's the same David who, 38 years later, is the Chief Operating Officer of Home Health, Hospice, and Quality at BAYADA. In a term paper titled "My Roots," written for his 10th grade social studies class at Moorestown Friends School in New Jersey, David summarized the history of his father's business and happily added that his birth "could possibly be the reason that my dad got the contract!" David's teacher noted "Great story!" and gave him an A. 🌿

told her that she would have to make the presentation. He drove my mom to Jefferson Hospital and, since my mom wasn't in labor yet, went to the office and worked from 1-6am getting the presentation notes together for his assistant. He spent the day at the hospital and the people at the presentation thought that it was great that a man put his family before his work and could possibly be the reason that my dad got the contract! *Great story!*

Many other things have changed since 1976. At the time, minimum wage was $2.35. My dad was just getting his business off of the ground and he deserved his hard earned success. His average day was very trying. He would wake up at 6:30 am to a very low temperature in order to save money. After having a breakfast of *Total* cereal he would walk to the bus stop and catch bus #9 and get dropped of at Market St. and walk to his First office at 1601 Walnut St. in Philadelphia. His office was in the Medical Arts building and he had a black desk and his files were kept very neat (another thing that has changed). He would leave the office between five and seven without ever eating lunch. He walked home from his bus stop, ate a simple dinner, and then continued his work until about midnight.

Over all, as a result of me being born, of course, my father thinks that 1976 was a very exciting year.

David's high school term paper described his dad's daily routine.

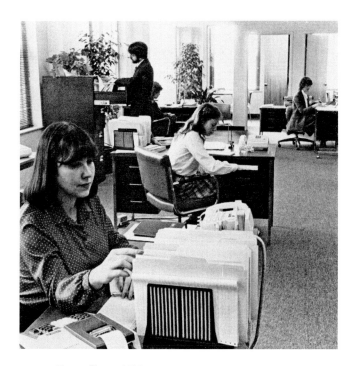

ABOVE: Bigger offices at 1315 Walnut Street meant the company was moving up in the world.

TOP RIGHT: The proprietary record system, BEARS, generated reams of printouts like this July 1980 "Cases by Supervisor" report.

RIGHT: First major contract: Philadelphia Corporation for Aging.

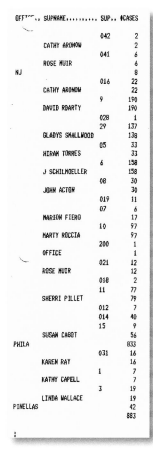

OFFICE,, SUPNAME..........	SUP,,	#CASES
	042	2
CATHY ARONOW		2
	041	6
ROSE MUIR		6
NJ		8
	016	22
CATHY ARONOW		22
	9	190
DAVID RDARTY		190
	028	1
	29	137
GLADYS SMALLWOOD		138
	05	33
HIRAM TORRES		33
	6	158
J SCHILMOELLER		158
	08	30
JOHN ACTON		30
	019	11
	07	6
MARION FIERO		17
	10	97
MARTY ROCCIA		97
	200	1
OFFICE		1
	021	12
ROSE MUIR		12
	018	2
	11	77
SHERRI PILLET		79
	012	7
	014	40
	15	9
SUSAN CABOT		56
PHILA		833
	031	16
KAREN RAY		16
	1	7
KATHY CAPELL		7
	3	19
LINDA WALLACE		19
PINELLAS		42
		883

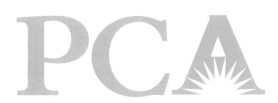

Getting busier

The PCA contract was a turning point—it doubled the business. In pre-computer days, that presented the company with operational challenges. For a while, binders were the answer. One binder contained client and case information; another was packed with employees' contact information. That system evolved to a more streamlined system of index cards.

Telephones were a lifeline. Office employees relied on an answering service run by live operators during non-office hours to relay after-hours calls. "Anytime we were out of the house, we would have to call in to the answering service to make sure there weren't any calls that came in," says Peggy.

Because Mark always had to stay on top of calls and be available to quickly resolve problems, he carried a large canvas tote bag with him everywhere. It was bursting at its seams with papers that listed contact information on home health aides and clients. For years, Mark himself was regularly on-call or would step in at the last minute. Once, in a pinch, he even turned to Little Jo—the second cousin who had inspired him to look into home care as a business opportunity—to fill in as a home health aide. She later became a full time live-in for BAYADA.

"I put my name on the list for callouts, and I'd visit clients periodically. When I showed up, they wouldn't know who I was," he observes.

Mark even bought a short white jacket and white pants to wear to visits. And he took 60 hours of home health aide training to become certified in 1984. Kathy (Kathaleen)

Telephone courtesy, then and now

Proper telephone manners may be falling by the wayside in our fast-paced society. But they are alive and well at BAYADA, where much business is still done by phone. From the start, the company has expected employees to "listen closely, show empathy, and respond to the needs of others" on every call. In 1977, Mark issued typewritten "Phone Rules" both to employees and the answering service that took calls after hours. ("Be patient," Rule 8 gently urges. "We have many elderly and emotionally upset callers.") Similarly, he had strict and specific expectations for his own children when they were young. David and Janice couldn't just answer "Hello," like many of their friends did. They were encouraged to include the family name: "Hello, Baiadas."

Almost 40 years later, similar guidelines are the focus of "Answering with the Stars," a company-created twist on TV's *Dancing with the Stars* that's accessible on the employee intranet. This fictitious reality radio show offers comical examples of the do's and don'ts of caller etiquette. In one example, the woman answering the phone sounds stressed and speaks in a clipped tone. The judge rules that she's giving the caller "The Hustle." When another woman answers in a friendly and professional way, she is praised for successfully using "The Front Line Fox Trot." As the program summarizes, "Answering like a Star is not easy. The best of the best work at it tirelessly."

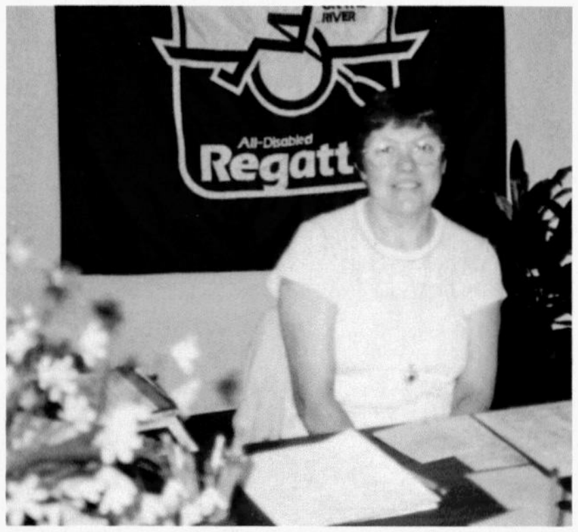

LEFT: Betty DeFeo was the company's beloved telephone voice in early years.

Reavy, who joined BAYADA in 1980, remembers his rationale. "Mark said, 'How am I going to tell people what's expected if I can't empathize or understand what they're doing?'" says Kathy, now Division Director in Moorestown, New Jersey. "That's totally him. I don't know that I've met anybody quite like him in my life."

From the beginning, reliability to clients and their families was a guiding principle. "We just didn't miss shifts," says Mark. "If we make a promise, we keep our commitment."

With client demands increasing, RN Home Health Care needed to quickly hire 100 more home health aides. This meant more office staff, too, as well as a bigger office in Philadelphia. That was the period when Mark moved his desk into the utility closet to accommodate the additional staff. "I remember it was a long, narrow closet. I got a stool," recounts Mark. "I just remember thinking, 'Hey, you've got to do what you've got to do.'" Peggy joined the business officially as well, leaving her job at the hospital in order to handle the company's payroll and accounting full time.

Boosting efficiency

To further help with office efficiency, Mark researched computerization. Large companies had used mainframes for decades, but systems for smaller businesses were scarce. Mark bought a small computer secondhand in 1977 and taught himself to program it. His younger brother Mel had a flair for technology. (Mel would go on to found a successful technology company that was bought by Hewlett-Packard in 2000.) With Mel's help, the company bought additional PCs

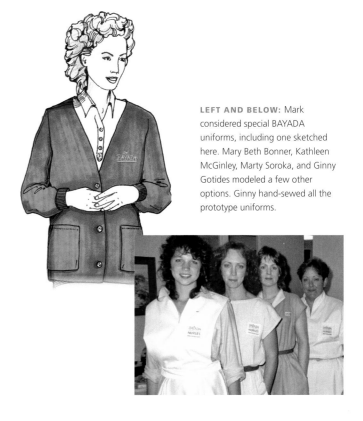

and adopted the Pick digital sharing system in 1978, an early innovation that allowed offices to share data.

Together, the brothers created a proprietary data management program playfully titled BEARS, which stands for BAYADA Exceptionally Advanced Record System—jokingly referred to by the brothers as the Baiada Exceptionally Awesome Record System. BEARS isn't graphically slick, but it is so robust that it has been updated through numerous versions and is still used. Colleen Thomas started in 1984 as the company's first computer programmer and has since moved up to Area Director of Information Services. She laughs when she remembers the company's first computer, nicknamed Arnold: "It was so big it occupied almost a whole room."

Colleen also has fond memories of the first fax machine. "A rep told us we would connect this giant thing to the phone line and then a payroll form would print out from offices. I practically shrieked, 'Get out! That's actually going to print out here?'" By the 1980s faxing would completely change the payroll process—among other areas—and dramatically save time. Employees and couriers no longer had to physically transport key documents between offices or worry that paycheck deliveries might be delayed by traffic jams. Home health aides and staff had earned those dollars and couldn't afford to wait for them.

While these technology steps might seem comical today, they were very innovative for their time. Even when Mark's company was small, he "thought big" and invested in systems that saved money and streamlined operations.

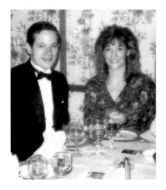

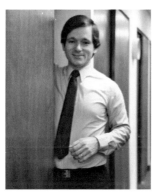

TOP: Mark and Linda Siessel in the early 1980s. "When I walked into that Philadelphia office, it was buzzing," Linda recalls. "So much energy and camaraderie! I picked up right away that it was okay to dream, okay to think very far out and work from your heart."

ABOVE: As office space grew tight, Mark actually moved his desk into a utility closet for a time.

LEFT AND BELOW: Mark considered special BAYADA uniforms, including one sketched here. Mary Beth Bonner, Kathleen McGinley, Marty Soroka, and Ginny Gotides modeled a few other options. Ginny hand-sewed all the prototype uniforms.

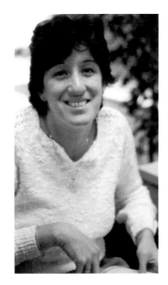

LEFT: Sherri Pillet in 1981. She was attracted to the company because "I had a degree in social work and wanted to make a difference to people. I also had some ambition and wanted to make some money. Not only could you blend both at this company, but you were expected to."

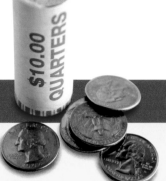

Big rolls of quarters and more: A short history of technology at BAYADA

Until the advent of pagers (also called beepers) in the 1980s and cell phones in the late 1990s, virtually all employees carried their hefty rolls of quarters and used pay phones to call into the office or answering service. Reaching employees at home was also challenging, especially in the days before the phone company introduced call-waiting services. If an employee's line was repeatedly busy, employees sometimes resorted to calling the telephone company operator and reporting a medical emergency. That allowed the operator to break into the employee's phone call in progress and put through RN Home Health Care's call. With luck, the employee would be able to cover the open shift.

Dialing those old rotary phones and feeding in the quarters took time. Back at the office, so did sorting out masses of curled pages from the fax machine—and eventually accessing the internet by connecting via a telephone modem that emitted a piercing screech.

Younger employees can be grateful that these antiquities have been replaced by PCs, laptops, smartphones, and tablets. When BAYADA is 100, will today's technologies seem as ancient as typewriters?

• **Beepers and pagers:** "A big technological breakthrough for doing on-call because you got alerted instead of having to periodically call in." —**Tom Mylet, Regional Director, Winston-Salem, North Carolina**

• **The Qwip® machine:** Made by Exxon, this was a pre-fax/phone line that used a spinning cylinder with thermal paper to transmit documents. The main users were national newspaper reporters, who used Qwip to file stories from afar while on tight deadlines. BAYADA would have been an early corporate user. "We had to buy a Qwip as a condition of a contract. Actually we had to buy two, so the contract holder could have one too." —**Tom Mylet**

• **Early mobile phones:** "We had probably a 10-pound phone on one side of our head and a five-pound pager on the other side of our body, plus a contraption that you wore on your head that wired you to the phone. Still we thought we had the coolest gear and the best job in the world!" —**Debra Magaraci, Director, Voorhees, New Jersey**

• **Desktop PCs and email:** Colleen Thomas hired someone in the mid-1980s just because the person had a home computer with email—revolutionary for the time. Email didn't come to BAYADA desktops until the 1990s. There was only one PC per office, so each person would check individual email every day on the main workstation. "Soon directors received a PC, then each office worker did. Today everyone in the company gets a PC, a laptop, or a tablet. And of course personal cell phones are in just about everyone's purse or pocket." — **Colleen Thomas, Area Director of Information Services, Langhorne, Pennsylvania** 🌿

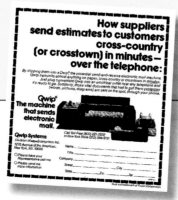

Putting a stake in the ground

The business grew fast, but not too fast. As with building the sea wall, Mark recognized that certain essentials cannot and should not be rushed. One of them, he believes, is interviewing. There was (and still is) thoughtful consideration of every job candidate. With a goal of fostering a warm, family-like environment for the company and for clients, Mark knew employees need to be extremely reliable and have a certain personality—a caring one. It's fairly easy to evaluate a person's skills and teach what needs to be learned; it's harder to evaluate and instill values like compassion and reliability. Although *The BAYADA Way* was still years away from being put into words, those core values were the qualities Mark prioritized.

A family friend once said to Mark, "If you stand for something, you'll attract people who feel the same way. You have to put a stake in the ground." This made innate sense. It was true of the U.S. Marines and the Jesuits, two entities that Mark admires. So he refined his process of finding like-minded professionals. Hiring the right people meant that those individuals became like family, because they shared RN Home Health Care's values. They bonded as they worked long hours together to answer calls and get shifts covered. They modeled the "community of compassionate caregivers" decades before that concept appeared in *The BAYADA Way.* Eventually, they became mentors to a new generation of employees, a vital role as the company grew. Mark knew hiring like-minded employees would make connections to last a lifetime, produce long-term careers at

BAYADA, and help him fulfill his vision of building a successful company while caring for others.

Bringing employees together for smiles, laughs, and stress reduction was a top priority. Just as the extended Baiada family regularly gathered for celebrations, the family of BAYADA employees loved to party, too. Any occasion will do: parties for recognizing employees, quarterly parties, holiday parties, billing records parties, summer parties, parties to celebrate marriages and births, and sometimes parties for no reason at all. "Work hard, play hard" was the rallying cry. In time, even the early training retreats would morph into today's weekend-long, party and recognition-rich Awards Weekend celebrations.

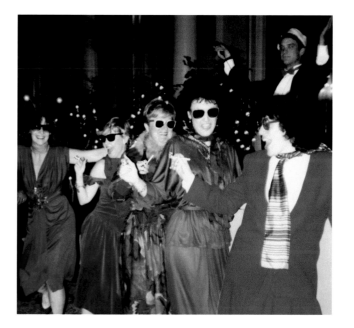

"Mark always had, and still has, a great sense of humor and a great way of making you feel like you're part of the family. You were part of what he wanted the company to become."

JOANNE WILSON, who started in 1982 as an Accounting Supervisor and is currently a Director working in the Home Care Technology office

LEFT: Linda Siessel, Kathy Moran Dempsey, Carole McMahon, Vicki Bolcar, and Marion Fiero getting into the swing of "work hard, play hard" in the 1980s.

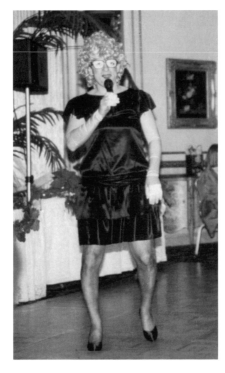

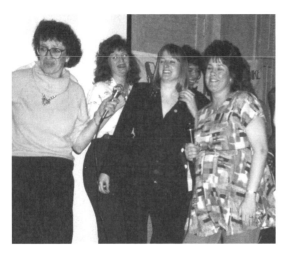

The fun generally includes skits and songs. While some company owners would never dream of looking silly in front of employees, Mark has always loved to perform at parties and events. What other corporate president has dressed up as various female characters (including a rock star), a caveman, a cowboy, and even one of the Blues Brothers? The nature of the skits, and the sometimes wacky costumes, spring from Mark's endlessly creative mind. "I always say Mark is a party looking for people," laughs Anita Palmer, Project Coordinator in charge of Awards Weekends.

The late 1970s were also joyful years for the Baiadas at home. Mark and Peggy welcomed their second child, Janice, in 1979. Juggling two small children while running a business wasn't easy, but fortunately the couple could reach out to local family members and their tight-knit work family to help.

ABOVE: Company celebrations provide Mark with plenty of chances to exercise the theatrical side of his personality.

ABOVE RIGHT: Karaoke fun in the mid-1980s with Marion Fiero, Mary DeScioli, Patricia Rohrer, and Colleen Thomas.

RIGHT: *The Muppet Movie* introduced Mark to his alter ego, Kermit the Frog, in 1979. The movie's theme has had a lasting effect on the company.

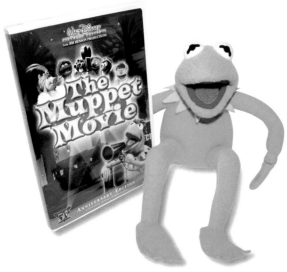

Meeting the Muppets

Another huge event of 1979 was *The Muppet Movie,* which made a profound impact on Mark. In the movie, Kermit the Frog is persuaded by an agent to go to Hollywood to pursue a career in the movies. Along the way, he meets a motley crew of characters with different talents but similar goals. They come together, resist villainous attempts to sell out to big commercial interests, and travel on Kermit's bus to pursue their common dreams. This struck a chord with Mark that has never stopped resonating: "We're just like them. We started small. And we have this bigger dream of 'going to Hollywood,' which for us means being the world's

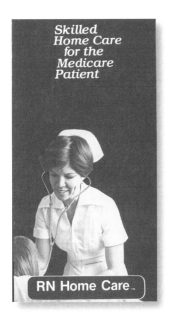

ABOVE: The company's first Medicare certification in 1980 proved to be a vital step forward.

RIGHT: Denise Pushnik, then Director of the Denver office, in 1982. Denver was office number 7. Expansion to Florida and Colorado signified key growth and a willingness to "think bigger."

most compassionate and trusted team of home health care professionals."

A big step toward the dream took place in 1980, when the company received its first Medicare certification, allowing it to care for many more clients. RN Home Health Care expanded its reach geographically and professionally, by adding such services as skilled nursing and pediatric care. By 1982, six offices had been opened—not just in suburban Philadelphia and New Jersey, but as far west as Denver, Colorado, and as far south as Pinellas Park, Florida. Accordingly, given the increased need for administrative space, the company moved its headquarters to Moorestown, New Jersey in 1982.

The move also allowed David Baiada, then age 6, to attend the historic Moorestown Friends School, whose campus is just a few blocks from the company's headquarters. MFS has since educated many young Baiada family members from preschool through grade 12. Founded by the Society of Friends in 1785, the school adheres to the Quaker values of simplicity, peace, integrity, community, equality, and stewardship. These values resonated strongly with Mark and have their counterparts in *The BAYADA Way.*

Business expansion continued, thanks to the company's solid relationships with clients and referral sources, its outstanding reputation, and its hardworking, reliable employees. Once a new office was opened, it would grow case by case—one week, one month, one year at a time. As offices grew, they typically split into smaller ones, sometimes offering just a single specialty, such as pediatric nursing or

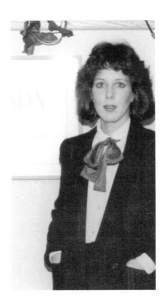

"I remember a terribly hot summer in Philadelphia in the early 1980s. We all felt bad because so few of our elderly clients had air conditioning. Many of them lived in difficult neighborhoods. They were afraid to open their windows because of the chance of crime. They were suffering. Mark bought fans for a whole group of them. Back then we didn't have the money, but Mark did it. It was sheer kindness. I remember thinking, that's what I want to be part of."

SHERRI PILLET, who started in 1980 and is now Division Director of Employee Relations, Burlington, New Jersey

Still getting the right people on the bus

While today's employment screenings are more formal, and the testing more scientific, the legacy of friendly but thorough evaluations is firmly entrenched. One example: Before Bruce Bosco was hired as Director of the Washington Township, New Jersey, office in 2008—a midcareer job transition—he spent almost two days in interviews. A few of those hours were with an industrial psychologist who flew in from Colorado. "BAYADA vetted the position really well," says Bruce, adding that the process allowed him to vet the company, too. "It actually drew me in more, because I saw the investment the company was making and how particular they were about who they were hiring." Now Bruce uses similar procedures when he hires: "We're still all about getting the right people on the bus." ❧

RIGHT: Job candidates are specifically evaluated on compassion, excellence, and reliability—the fundamental values of *The BAYADA Way.*

BAYADA Employment Application - Insert

PLEASE PRINT

INTERVIEW WRITE-UP

Date	Position		Prospect #	Employee #

Applicant Name				Pay Required

Please rate the applicant on the following (see reverse for interpretative guidelines):

_____ Presence   _____ Experience   _____ Comprehension   _____ Attitude   _____ Skills   _____ Maturity

RATING KEY: 5 Very Much Above Standard   4 Above Standard   3 Meets Standard   2 Below Standard   1 Very Much Below Standard

Evaluations
Be sure to evaluate prior work experience, test and skill results, appropriateness for BAYADA Home Health Care, and overall interview conclusions.

Prior Work Experience

Test and Skill Results

Appropriateness for BAYADA

Compassion

Excellence

Reliability

Overall Interview Conclusions

FOLLOW-UP NOTES

Interviewer	Date Interviewed	Approved By	Date

0-378 5/11 © BAYADA Home Health Care, 2011

personal care services from home health aides. The company still encountered occasional resistance in a field dominated by nonprofit competitors. While this was frustrating to Mark, he used it as motivation: "We're just going to give better service and be more responsive." Like Kermit in *The Muppet Movie,* he saw life as being bigger than one's own pond. Within the world of home care, BAYADA was forging a "rainbow connection," a reference to Kermit's song about his quest to follow his dreams.

Intensive and unorthodox interviews

Job candidates are often amazed at the length and intensity of the BAYADA hiring process. Long before the company introduced *The BAYADA Way* as a screening tool, Mark and others sought to "get the right people on the bus." Their methods have sometimes taken potential employees by surprise.

At Kathy (Kathaleen) Reavy's initial interview in 1980, for example, she couldn't help but notice a novelty walnut on the president's desk that read Head Nut. "This is going to be interesting," she thought. She and Mark quickly discovered similar Catholic school backgrounds and large families. Their conversation went on for three hours.

Eventually Mark mentioned a job, saying in broad terms that he wanted to open and staff an office in New Jersey. Then he asked if Kathy had seen *The Muppet Movie.* She replied, "Yes, it was a nice little movie." Mark practically jumped out of his chair, educating her on the point of the film. "I'm sitting there very wide-eyed by now," reflects Kathy. "Finally Mark said, 'So, you want to be a Muppet?' I said, 'I've got to get back to you.'"

ABOVE: Tom Mylet was surprised to learn that his handwritten application letter was analyzed by a graphologist. In the early years, Mark used handwriting analysis as one of several tools to assess personal and professional traits. Tom's writing passed muster and opened the door to a long and satisfying career.

BELOW: Urged by her dad to "steer clear" of a company run by a fervent Muppet fan, Kathy Reavy took the job offer anyhow. She's now in her fourth decade at BAYADA.

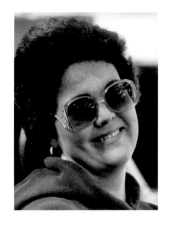

Kathy's dad urged her to "steer clear of this kook," but her mom said "give it a try." After a second interview, which lasted a mere two hours, Kathy started working as a Staff Supervisor. Just three months later, she was promoted to Director of the first office in New Jersey. Today, Kathy is the Division Director of Benefits and Employee Claims and Safety.

Recently degreed as a social worker in 1982, Tom Mylet answered a newspaper ad for a Staff Supervisor (today's Client Services Manager). It called for a résumé and a one-page, handwritten letter about the applicant's choice of social work as a career. Tom sent both and got the job. "I was here probably three years before anyone even admitted to me that the letter was submitted for handwriting analysis," laughs Tom, now Regional Director of Adult State Services in Winston-Salem, North Carolina.

Learning to listen better

Creating a culture of camaraderie helped temper the frenetic pace of a growing business and reduce the stress of work that routinely involves illness, accidents, and death. It also had the subtle effect, as David Baiada later noted, of casting a "halo effect" on relationships in the offices. People who played and laughed together built a sense of trust and friendship that got them through tough times, both personally and professionally. New colleagues were welcomed and made to feel like family.

In turn, the solid relationships helped employees listen better, a vital business skill. "When a client calls you, you're there, fully attentive to what they're saying," says Mark.

"Mark's got something to teach the world. He really does. His talent is naturally where it is, he's in the right place at BAYADA, but I often think he should be teaching in one of those prestigious business schools like Wharton or Harvard."

ANNA ANDERSON,
who started in 1987 and is now Client Services Manager in Morristown, New Jersey (Anna is also the first recipient of The Linda Siessel Award for Excellence in Client Services Leadership)

RIGHT: The company newsletter underwent a few changes of name and format before it became the *BAYADA Bulletin* of today. But it always blended professional information with employee news.

1979

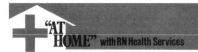

1988

1998

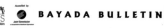

2004

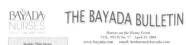

2009

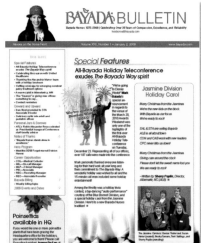

2015

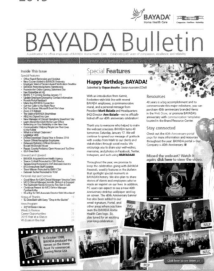

"You have to listen really carefully, try to connect with them, and try to understand the total situation. If you make a promise, you keep that commitment. Sometimes we need to help each other to always listen closely, always let our smiles be seen and felt even on a bad day, because you have to do this reliably. It is easy to get a little snippy when you are under pressure. When you are working in home care, you have to realize that the situations your clients are facing are extremely difficult—something they never wanted for themselves or their family. You have to empathize and let that pressure motivate you to do a better job."

Kindness toward clients and kindness toward employees were one and the same. Mark knew that committed employees were the foundation of the company's success. In fact, early on, he even supported an office manager who wanted to move south to open the Pinellas Park, Florida, office. That was the first of many offices opened by trustworthy employees with a hankering to relocate. Not all of these offices survived, but most did, and they created a pattern in which company growth sprang from real human relationships as well as research and data analysis.

As companies and families get bigger and start to disperse, past rituals can get lost. Mark took pains not to let that happen. To keep people connected, the company launched the *RN Home Health Care Newsletter*. It wasn't fancy, more like a letter from home. That was the idea—to keep employees in different offices informed of news, community service efforts, and billings, as well as engagements, marriages, births, and passings. Each issue ended with a heart-tugging thank-you note from a client or a client's

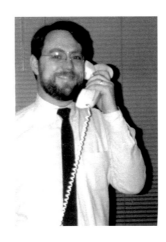

ABOVE: Tom Mylet was one of several early Philadelphia-area employees who remain with BAYADA at its fortieth anniversary. Tom went on to open and build the company's operations in North Carolina.

BELOW: His early name badge was made on a machine at Headquarters. Making those name badges was an occasional after-school task for young David Baiada.

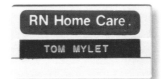

family. The newsletter evolved into the more robust *BAYADA Bulletin,* which transitioned from print publication to e-distribution in 2000. To this day, the weekly *BAYADA Bulletin* remains jam-packed with employee submissions.

A new name and other turning points

With growth came the decision to change the company name. RN Home Health Care had been tweaked a few times, to RN Home Care and RN Health Services, during the early years. Mark now wanted to solidly differentiate the company in a rapidly growing market. He is a great believer in consensus, so he asked employees for ideas and opinions. Some of his own choices, he admits, were "really out there."

If Mark had had his way, the company might have been renamed Hygieia, for the Greek goddess of health; or Little Nurses for Home Care, after the Little Sisters of the Poor; or Oak or Elm or Maple, for solidity. Fortunately, wisdom prevailed. As Mark explains, "Finally someone said, 'Let's call it Baiada.' And I thought, 'That's a little prideful.' Then I thought, well, people will know there's somebody behind this company who takes responsibility for it. But there's the spelling problem. I've lived with it. I grew up with it. I know how people can never get Baiada right. So someone suggested we just change the spelling." The phonetic spelling of Baiada would make it easier to spell and pronounce. That solution had worked well for the Bloch family, who founded H&R Block, the Toyoda family, who founded Toyota Motor Company, and Marcel Bich, the Frenchman who invented Bic pens.

"We are a family"

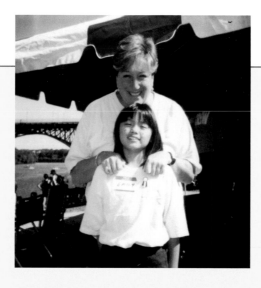

Every family has its own set of values, spoken and unspoken. *The BAYADA Way* places its values front and center. Employees follow them, live them every day, and build connections that encourage a family-like atmosphere at work. Happily, that spirit often extends to employees' children, who absorb lasting lessons in compassion, excellence, and reliability.

At the annual adaptive rowing competition, the BAYADA Regatta, as well as other charitable events, children of employees pitch in and volunteer. "I always brought my kids to the Regatta because it gave them an opportunity to help, and also to see what people with disabilities can be capable of," says Colleen Thomas.

Through company events and close ties, children of BAYADA employees got to know each other, too. In the early years, Director Joanne Wilson's daughter babysat Janice and David Baiada in the summertime. "We are not just co-workers. We are not just staff," says Wilson, who's been with the company since 1982. "We are a family."

Sherri Pillet, who joined in 1980, appreciates that all-in-the-BAYADA-family feeling. In 1995, while preparing to adopt a child from China, she knew the day her daughter's picture was to be faxed to headquarters. "I will never forget it," says Sherri, now Division Director of Employee Relations in Burlington, New Jersey. "When the fax started to come in downstairs, Mark jumped up and ran upstairs to gather all the employees who were sitting there and then ran around to get others, so they would all be there to support me."

The office took on a charged atmosphere, filled with the kind of tingling, lump-in-the-throat anticipation found only at joyous events that are poised to change a person's life forever. When the grainy image of the baby's face emerged from 10,000 miles away, the group oohed, aahed, shrieked, and didn't hide their tears. They instantly became a roomful of loving godmothers and godfathers. Each one of them still remembers that moment as if it were yesterday. "Everyone was so genuinely excited and caring. I remember thinking how incredibly lucky I was," Sherri emphasizes. At BAYADA's fortieth anniversary, her baby has grown up to become a Drexel University undergraduate.

Living by *The BAYADA Way* offers a powerful example to kids, some of whom decide to become BAYADA employees themselves. "I've raised my children to help people, to thank people for doing a great job, to care about people, and to make a difference," says Colleen. "My kids are very kind and caring. We think *The BAYADA Way* is a really wonderful way to live your whole life." 🌿

ABOVE: Sherri Pillet and her daughter, Emily, volunteering at the 2004 BAYADA Regatta.

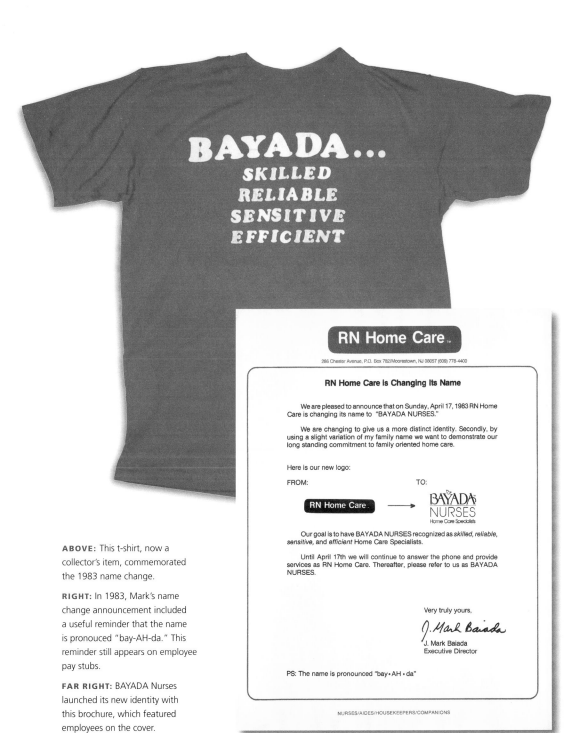

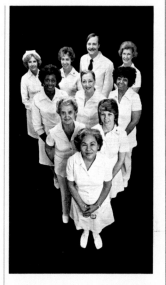

ABOVE: This t-shirt, now a collector's item, commemorated the 1983 name change.

RIGHT: In 1983, Mark's name change announcement included a useful reminder that the name is pronouced "bay-AH-da." This reminder still appears on employee pay stubs.

FAR RIGHT: BAYADA Nurses launched its new identity with this brochure, which featured employees on the cover.

In 1983, the official name became BAYADA Nurses. Its tagline was Skilled, Reliable, Sensitive, and Efficient. "I always did like efficient," Mark says.

As the company's new identity gained momentum, life at home for Mark and Peggy was changing. Over time, the two drifted apart. Peggy would move to Philadelphia in 1984, while Mark, David, and Janice stayed in their home in Moorestown. Mark and Peggy made good on their promise to put the children's needs first. The marriage ended amicably. Peggy continued to work at the company until 1987.

"Growing up, I saw some of my friends' parents getting divorced, and it was really bad. They were contentious. And then it occurred to me, even as a young kid, that, 'Wow, my parents still get along. This is special, and I'm really lucky,'" says daughter Janice Lovequist, who is currently Manager, *The BAYADA Way* Team.

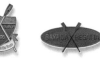

1989   1990   1991   1992   1993   1994   1995   1996   1997   1998   1999   2000   2001

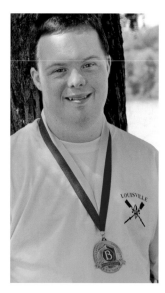

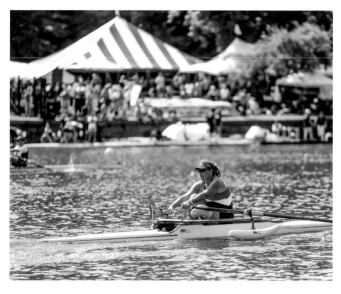

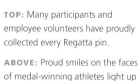

TOP: Many participants and employee volunteers have proudly collected every Regatta pin.

ABOVE: Proud smiles on the faces of medal-winning athletes light up each Regatta.

ABOVE RIGHT: Athlete Margaret Rajnic from the Capital Rowing Club.

RIGHT: At the 1995 Regatta were Mark, Philadelphia City Councilman Michael Nutter (later Mayor), Ron Castille, Bob Hardegan, and Mayor Ed Rendell (later Governor). Front: adaptive rowing pioneer Isabel Bohn and her granddaughter Anya Leiby.

BELOW: This signed oar was a gift to Mark from the PRPD, thanking him for his support of adaptive rowing and sponsorship of the annual BAYADA Regatta.

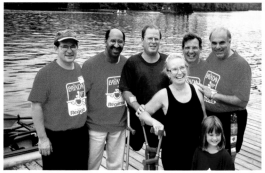

Birth of the BAYADA Regatta

One of the wedding engagements reported in the *RN Home Health Care Newsletter* indirectly led to the conception of the BAYADA Regatta. The Baiadas had attended an employee wedding where they met Dan Fanelli, a technical advisor and coach at the Philadelphia Rowing Program for the Disabled, known as PRPD (later renamed the Philadelphia Adaptive Rowing club, or PAR). Dan had talked passionately about a competitive rowing regatta for athletes with disabilities that had been held on the Schuylkill River, and Mark had been fascinated. The Freedom on the River Regatta had begun independently in 1981; with sponsorship from the company, it debuted as the BAYADA Regatta in 1983. Mark saw the Regatta as an opportunity to help people and to support the company's recent name change.

The annual event is still going strong, attracting rowers from across the country and around the globe to experience the thrill of adaptive rowing. Using single and double shells (a long, narrow rowing boat designed for racing) adapted for stability, the Regatta accommodates all levels of athletes and abilities, from beginners to Paralympians. Persevering athletes with disabilities like quadriplegia, cerebral palsy, multiple sclerosis, and blindness train throughout the year for the big event.

Just how big? At BAYADA's fortieth anniversary, the Regatta has grown to become one of the largest all-adaptive competitive rowing events in the world, and the longest running.

"Competitors say that adaptive rowing has changed their lives," Mark says. "After you have an injury, you get down and depressed. Everything can look hopeless. But when you

2002   2003   2004   2005   2006   2007   2008   2009   2010   2011   2012   2013   2014

get into adaptive rowing, there is a camaraderie with other rowers. You leave your wheelchair on the dock and you're just like everyone else. It gives people who may have lost hope or confidence the opportunity to socialize, compete, and feel accomplished."

Mark has been deeply involved with the Regatta since its infancy, overseeing its project management. BAYADA hosts a "Jolly Up" event the night before, which includes registration along with a festive open bar and food for all the rowers, and a dinner following the race day.

Not only does the Regatta live on, but BAYADA often donates a shell to either a new adaptive rowing program or one competing in the Regatta for the first time. This generosity has inspired rowing programs to form in different parts of the country, including Louisville, Kentucky, and Stockton, California.

Financial support is only part of the story. The event couldn't happen without the team of BAYADA volunteers, who start planning and fundraising a year in advance. They organize the setup, cleanup, and food for the rowers and their families, as well as the entertainment, which includes a DJ, face painters, and crafts for kids. On event day, the first volunteers arrive at dawn. One of them is Facilities Manager Ann Schaller, who every year drives the U-Haul with all Regatta supplies to the St. Joseph University Boathouse.

"It's actually pretty funny to see me driving a big truck," says Ann. "But helping at the Regatta is truly one of my favorite things. It's an awesome experience." She and dozens of other BAYADA people—and their families—pitch in until the event ends some 14 hours later.

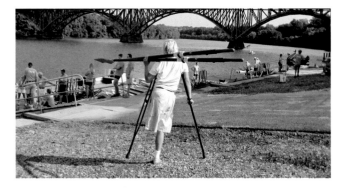

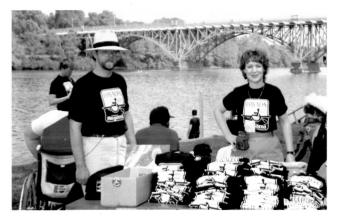

Reaching out to the community through the Regatta is just one example of BAYADA's "giving back" spirit and the company's commitment to community. Such service is worthwhile for its own sake—"We believe in providing community service where we live and work" is one of the beliefs articulated in *The BAYADA Way*—and is also part of relationship-building. Entire offices as well as individual employees regularly volunteer in fundraisers and benefits for clients or foundations supporting client diagnoses.

"Some companies might sponsor something like the Regatta in their early years and quit once they became prominent. The fact that Mark has continued it for more than 33 years is just one example of how genuine he is."

MAUREEN WRIGHT,
who started in 1983 and
is now Area Director of
Philadelphia Specialized
Contracts

ABOVE: Patty Michaud, a longtime BAYADA Regatta athlete.

LEFT: Tom Mylet and Marty Soroka volunteering at the first annual BAYADA Regatta in 1983.

BELOW: Shells named in honor of Mark and Isabel Bohn.

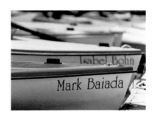

"When you work here, the Baiadas become everybody's family. The support of the Baiada family is never-ending."

GINNY GOTIDES, who started in 1982 and is a retired Division Director

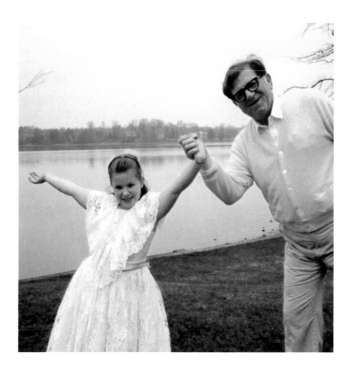

ABOVE: Aided by Grandpop Larry Baiada, Janice shows off the lacy First Communion dress that two employees gently encouraged her to choose.

Work, family, and the future

Life was beyond busy for Mark as the primary caretaker of two growing children and the leader of a demanding business, yet he remained unruffled. His work family often stepped in to help. BAYADA's ingrained philosophies of "all-hands-on-deck" and "family first" embraced the kids without fuss. David and Janice often spent late afternoons at the office. They'd stuff payroll envelopes and sometimes play in the supply closet among the reams of paper and pens.

Many employees treated the Baiada kids like their own, cheering for their sports achievements and helping them blow out candles on birthday cakes. One of Janice's favorite memories is when long-time employees Rita Rollo and Margaret Malloy took her shopping for her First Holy Communion dress. She tentatively zeroed in on a very ornate, over-the-top style covered in lace—a far cry from the simpler styles she was accustomed to when shopping with her dad—and was thrilled when Rita and Margaret praised her choice. Thinking of that "girly" dress still prompts a wide smile from Janice: "Oh, that dress! You wouldn't believe it. There was definitely a lot going on with that dress!" She laughs, "I just loved it!"

David enjoyed plenty of encouragement and love, too. He remembers that when he was about five years old, he wanted to sell pumpkins. He tried growing some in the backyard, but they withered from lack of sunlight. So his parents drove him to a farmer's market to buy some. David resold them to BAYADA employees who happily paid his slightly marked-up price and didn't care that the pumpkins weren't homegrown. "It was my first entrepreneurial experience," he jokes.

It wasn't unusual for David and Janice to be the last children picked up from extended day care at Moorestown Friends School. "That wasn't necessarily a bad thing," says David. "It was just what it was. I don't know that I was able to draw the connection at the time that things were busy at work for my dad. I think in hindsight, we were very shielded from what was happening at BAYADA."

Sometimes Mark's father, Grandpop Larry, would pick them up and care for them at his house. As he did with his own kids, Larry reinforced the Baiada family ethics of working hard, showing love, and having fun. He'd encourage David and Janice to do chores or to go outside, run around, and "blow the stink off," as he would often say. He knew they needed rigorous exercise for their health and happiness. It didn't hurt Grandpop's sanity, either.

Despite Mark's personal and professional responsibilities, he carved out time to coach his kids' soccer teams. He ate dinner with David and Janice every single night. As months and then years passed, Janice and David adjusted well to life with divorced parents and a father who worked a lot. "I don't remember ever thinking I missed out on this or that because my dad had to work," says David. "It was amazing. His time was definitely stretched, but he never showed it was stressing him out, or that Janice or I would have to make sacrifices to accommodate for it."

After a dozen years in business, Mark could look back and feel deep satisfaction. At age 40, he had realized his

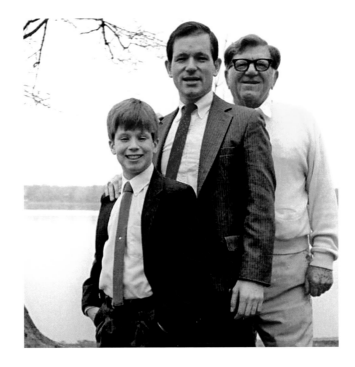

LEFT: David, Mark, and Larry Baiada on Janice's Communion Day. Each generation has carried forward the "family first" philosophy integral to the Baiadas and BAYADA.

dream: to launch a successful company that made a difference to others. He was the founding father of BAYADA, whose employees interacted like family and who cared compassionately for clients and their families. He was the father of two happy children who were thriving at school and at home. He was a good son and a caring brother to siblings who were making their own marks on the world.

But while Mark likes to measure success, he doesn't rest on past laurels or stand still. Always forward-looking, he had a feeling that something major might happen soon—at BAYADA and in his life. And it did.

Longevity and Loyalty: The 25-Year Club

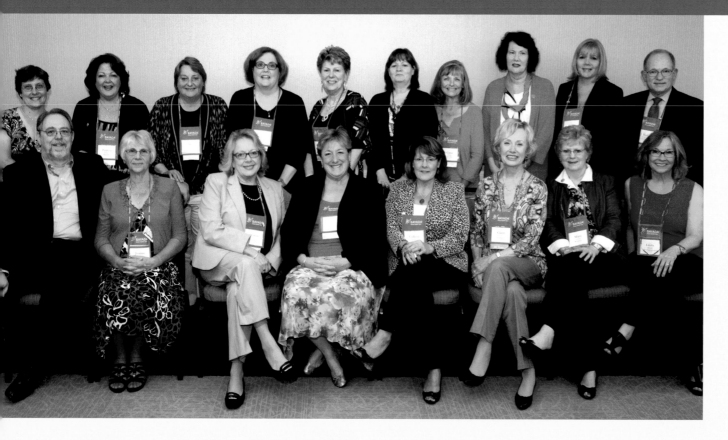

BACK ROW: Patricia Vattilana, Patricia Watson, Anne Johnson, Kathy Reavy, Anna Anderson, Mary DeScioli, Carol Elliott, Maureen Wright, Grace Dugan, Mark Baiada

FRONT ROW: Tom Mylet, Joanne Wilson, Marion Fiero, Sherri Pillet, Colleen Thomas, Ginger McCulloch, Marty Soroka, Linda Siessel

NOT PICTURED: Ann Baiada, Clare Gallagher, Ginny Gotides, Maryann Kinsley, Carole McMahon, Ann Miller, Judy Reinke, Rita Rollo, Cheryl Seiler, Linda Thomas, Ellen Wiest

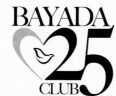

The average time an American employee stays in a job is 4.6 years. But don't tell that to the official BAYADA 25-Year Club. At the company's fortieth anniversary, this group includes more than two dozen people, some who joined as early as 1978. Most have enjoyed a succession of jobs within BAYADA, which offers the best of both worlds—opportunity and job security—to employees with an entrepreneurial bent.

Ask members of the club or any of the decades-long employees or retirees why they stay, and they'll likely say it's the unwavering, caring leadership of Mark and Ann Baiada; the company's tangible values; and its family feel.

"Mark started the company with an example of doing the right thing and giving the best service," says Carole McMahon, Division Director in Haverford, Pennsylvania, who joined in

1980. "Knowing the difference you can make in someone's life is kind of contagious, and that's why I've stayed."

Marty Soroka knows a thing or two about longtime employees. At the company since 1978, a loyal, honest, cherished employee herself, she rattles off examples of office and field employees who have been with BAYADA for decades. One aide, she notes, worked with the same client throughout her 20-year history (the client stayed with the company for 30 years). Another aide was hired at age 65 and worked steadily until age 85. Currently, at least 25 aides on her workforce are over age 65 with at least two aides still covering shifts in their 80s—with energy, compassion, and a keen understanding of what her elderly clients are thinking and feeling.

Another reason for long-term loyalty? The bonds among coworkers just get stronger with every passing year. "I think anybody who's spent any time working at BAYADA or with Mark knows that connection," adds Marty, who is Division Director of the Personal Care Assistant Office in Philadelphia. "The support we need on a daily basis from peers—like when you're having a bad day or you just need help—it's always there. It's our atmosphere, and it all comes from what Mark started back in 1975." ❧

The 25-Year Club in Chronological Order

Members	Start Date	Current Title
Mark Baiada	January 1975	President/Founder
Martha Soroka	January 1978	Division Director
Marion Fiero	November 1979	Division Director
Sherri Pillet	March 1980	Division Director
Kathaleen Reavy	September 1980	Division Director
Carole McMahon	October 1980	Division Director
Linda Siessel	October 1980	Chief Operating Officer, HCS
Joanne Wilson	February 1982	Director
Maryann Kinsley	April 1982	Office Manager
Ginny Gotides	May 1982	Division Director (Retired)
Thomas Mylet	August 1982	Regional Director
Maureen Wright	June 1983	Area Director
Ginger McCulloch	August 1983	Clinical Manager
Cheryl Seiler	October 1983	Administrative Assistant
Colleen Thomas	February 1984	Area Director
Judy Reinke	April 1984	Administrative Coordinator
Rita Rollo	September 1984	Administrative Assistant
Anne Johnson	November 1984	Division Director
Patricia Vattilana	December 1984	Medicare Case Manager
Mary DeScioli	February 1986	Recruiter
Carol Elliott	October 1986	Help Desk Analyst
Patricia Watson	March 1987	Division Director
Anna Anderson	November 1987	Client Services Manager
Grace Dugan	June 1988	Associate Director
Clare Gallagher	January 1989	Clinical Support Associate (Retired)
Ann Baiada	February 1989	Director
Ellen Wiest	November 1989	Clinical Manager
Ann Miller	January 1990	Clinical Educator
Linda Thomas	January 1990	Client Services Manager

CHAPTER TWO

Transformations
"Be Led by Our Hearts"

RIGHT: A sampling of thank-you letters from grateful clients and employees from over the years.

Mr. J. Mark Baiada
Home Health Care

Dear Mr. Baiada,

We were most fortunate to have three employees of Bayada: two physical therapists and one occupational therapist.

We always were informed of the days and time we could expect them, which was most helpful to us. Their alloted time was reasonable.

We would highly recommend ~yada Home Health Care to anyone ~ing this kind of care.

~ayada Home Health Care
1777 Sentry Parkway West
Dublin Hall Ste 101

Att: Mr. J. Mark Baiada,
Dear Mr. Baiada,

Re: Sharon

Sharon discharged me from Therapy yesterday I have to let you know That she is one of the most professional women I have met. She called The day before she came, To confirm the Time - she was never late, she helped me To "Walk Again." You should be very proud to have an employee such as she.

I know of what I speak. I was an R.N. for 51 years before retirement~

~e joined Bayada nurses last Dec. and have loved every minute of it. I never realized home care could be so much fun. I will never go back to a Doctors office again!

My point in this Letter is to tell you about the wonderful professional women that I interact with on a frequent basis. The team at the Morristown, NJ office are terrific. They are professional, dedicated, caring and so hard working, and I know their job is not easy. I'm the kind of person who loves to give credit to he~

And, finally, you definitely need to know of Sharon is from New Jersey, she needs no explanation. Sharon was the weeks of caring and it was Sharon who was there the fin non-stop, not sleeping or eating, just supporting my sister, n nurse, and our Mother. The caring details that Sharon tende Mother were far too many to mention. She is a goldmine of mother was especially fond of Sharon as she reminded her c Sharon used every detail of that insight to assist Mom in sm really facing death in the face. There are no words to descri

Mr. Baiada, do you interview in Heaven for these women? trying time in our lives and the last of our Mother's life. Mc consistent genuine ardent care provided by these four wome a doubt a gift from God to us all. I hope you meet each pers acknowledge their extreme skill and ability.

By the way, even your accounting staff are pleasant. I have of mind to complete the accounting needs my Mother's esta our payment much later than it should have been sent. I wil Bayada Home Care Specialists with the highest esteem and appropriate persons and places. My experience with our Mc death will probably launch a reactive and resource filled alli assure you that Bayada will always be mentioned with the p ~leasant nature your people truly have earned as a reputatic

Dear Mark Baiada,

I am writing this letter to let you know that my husband John and I, his wife, Jean are more than satisfied with Kathy, our Hero on the Home Front. If you were to have a model for Bayada nurses, Kathy should be it. She is caring, thoughtful, knowledgeable, helpful and even though she gets things done so efficiently and promptly, she is never in a rush. It always seemed as though my husband were the only patient she had to see that day. We thank the Lord for Kathy and Bayada nurses.

"We are nice all the time.
It's not all that easy to be nice all the time."
CRIS TOSCANO, DIVISION DIRECTOR

BELOW: Ann Claffey Baiada brought transformative change to the Baiadas and BAYADA.

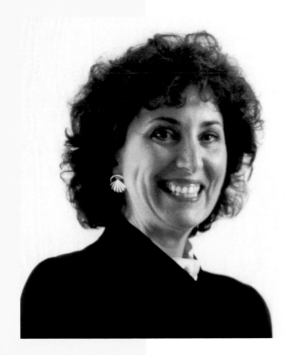

I n his quest for BAYADA Nurses to help more people, Mark began to think about adding rehabilitation services. He knew that rehab was a demanding specialty, one that couldn't be undertaken lightly. In 1988, he discussed the idea with a colleague who encouraged him to talk to a friend of hers—Ann Claffey, RN, CRRN (Certified Registered Rehabilitation Nurse). The mutual friend described Ann as a hardworking dynamo who had built a successful rehabilitation nursing program for a BAYADA competitor in the Philadelphia area.

"Ann had a reputation of doing great clinical management and getting all the rehab business, all the referrals," says Mark. "So I wanted to talk to her and possibly hire her." The two met in December 1988 and discovered they had a lot in common. At the end of the meeting, Mark asked Ann to join BAYADA as the first rehab nurse on staff and to launch a rehabilitation nursing program.

A single mother with three daughters—Jaclyn, then age 12; Kelli, age 10; and Christin, age 4—Ann had been working two part-time jobs and one full-time

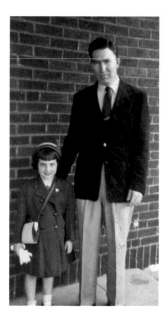
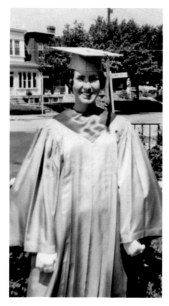
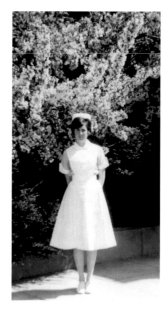

TOP ROW: Ann and her father, James Claffey. The Claffeys lived in Germantown, a working-class area in Northwest Philadelphia.

This happy graduate of Cardinal Dougherty High School was inducted into the school's Hall of Fame in 2003.

Ann as a second-year nursing student in 1967. She earned her RN degree at Abington Memorial Hospital School of Nursing in Abington, Pennsylvania, which honored her in 2014 with its Hall of Fame Award.

RIGHT: Edith Claffey, Ann's mother, was a charge nurse (shift supervisor) at Germantown Hospital. Edith's love of her profession helped inspire Ann and her sister to pursue nursing careers.

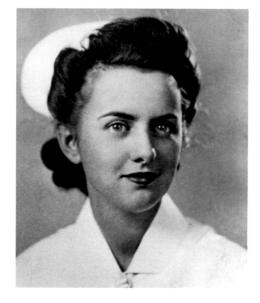

job to make ends meet. Like Mark, she knew the value of a close, extended family. She and her girls had lived with Ann's parents in Oreland, near Philadelphia, since Ann's divorce in 1985. Nursing was in her blood; her mother and sister Carolyn were nurses, too.

As they spoke, Ann asked Mark some hard, practical questions. She had philosophical differences with her full-time employer and was ready for a change. But changing jobs is always a risk, especially for a single parent and breadwinner. Ann is an excellent judge of character, and her intuition told her that she could trust Mark's promise. She also knew of the company's solid reputation. Determining that she would have a brighter future with BAYADA, with an opportunity to build a specialty that could make a significant difference, she said "yes."

In January 1989, Ann joined BAYADA. To remain near her family, she worked from the office in Willow Grove, Pennsylvania. Mark's willingness to let employees work in locations that make the most sense for them and their families—not necessarily for the company—is yet another example of his "family first" ethic in action.

Ann's family values

Ann's childhood had a lot in common with Mark's, except that she grew up on the Pennsylvania side of the Delaware River in an Irish family, not an Italian one. Ann was deeply influenced by her parents. Her father, James Claffey, worked as a federal government supply officer. She was proud that her dad was the only one in the neighborhood who wore a suit and tie to work every day and carried a briefcase.

James regularly volunteered at the Immaculate Conception Catholic Church in Germantown (Philadelphia) and at the parochial school the young Claffeys attended, lending a helping hand wherever needed. He was also a member of the Knights of Columbus, a Catholic service organization. Ann's mom, Edith, was a charge nurse (shift supervisor) in the emergency room at Germantown Hospital. "She was one tough woman and didn't take any nonsense from anyone," Ann says fondly.

Edith was one of the few full-time working mothers in the neighborhood. She worked the night shift, hurried home, and went to bed after her four children left for school. They walked home for lunch, so she'd wake up, feed them, and grab a few more hours of rest before the school day ended. She certainly wasn't a typical 1950s wife and mom. But she was revered because, as Ann recalls, "she would do anything for anyone. She was the first woman, the first person, anybody in the neighborhood called if there was a problem, if someone was sick, if someone got hurt, if someone had a tick in their head—anything at all. My mother would go over and decide, yes, this one has appendicitis and needs to get to the hospital. Yes, this one needs an enema. My mother probably gave an enema to half the people in our neighborhood." Not surprisingly, Ann adds, "some of the local kids were scared of her."

When a local family was quarantined due to a case of meningitis, Edith coordinated meals for them. If someone on the block needed a babysitter, Edith offered Ann's services. If they needed help with food shopping, she'd lend a hand or volunteer one of her kids to do it. Helping others was as

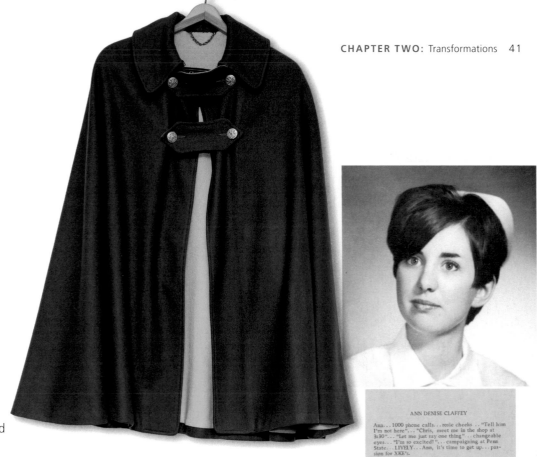

ANN DENISE CLAFFEY

Ann...1000 phone calls...rosie cheeks.."Tell him I'm not here"..."Chris, meet me in the shop at 3:30"..."Let me just say one thing"...changeable eyes..."I'm so excited!"...campaigning at Penn State...LIVELY...Ann, it's time to get up...passion for XKE's.

White cap and white shoes

One of Ann's most vivid memories is watching her mother in the mornings when she got home from work and the kids were getting ready for school. As tired as she must have been after eight hours in the emergency room, Edith always took time to polish her white shoes and delicately put away her nursing cap and nursing pins. It's no surprise that Ann and her sister, Carolyn, became nurses. "It impressed us as a wonderful profession," Ann says. 🌿

ABOVE: Ann has carefully preserved her first nursing cape and her very first RN cap, the same cap she wore in her yearbook photo. "My personal belief is that the day the hospital nurses took their caps off, we shot ourselves in the foot," Ann says. "I think that was a bad change. Just like the military wears their uniforms, we wore ours. Uniforms and caps stand for something. You know who you're looking at."

"Ann Baiada is one of my heroes in this organization. She's a nurse's nurse. A number of years ago when I was rolling out the mentoring program, she came up to me one day and tapped me on the shoulder and said, 'You are going to go places, my friend.' It was such a lovely thing. Nothing provoked it. It fueled my fire to want to grow, grow, grow in the company. It was a compliment that had a life beyond the compliment."

MARIE BLESSINGTON, RN, who started in 1985 as a home health aide and is now Director of Clinical Leadership Development, Moorestown, New Jersey

natural as breathing in the Claffey household. "My parents were very, very giving people and always there for others. They had strong social and charitable consciences," says Ann. "It was just part of our growing up—to give back and to do good things."

Ann makes waves

Ann immediately knew she had made the right move. "Very quickly, I found the difference amazing because BAYADA always was about quality and caring," says Ann. "It started at the top and still remains at the top. And it felt more like being with your family every day, working on something together, than coming to a job."

Before long, however, Ann noticed a few administrative inefficiencies. Because she was supervising rehabilitation cases in four different offices, she soon discovered that each office had its own set of forms and way of organizing care. She admits that BAYADA was providing excellent care at the time, but the lack of standardization didn't meet her approval.

"After about three weeks, I finally went to Mark," she says. "I was a big pain in the neck. I said, 'I don't understand how you think I can supervise properly when every office functions differently.' So it was around that time that a few other nursing supervisors and I decided to standardize our forms. Some people weren't thrilled about it. It was a lot easier just to fill out a little form than it was to comply with all these regulations and standards." She appreciated that she didn't have to tiptoe around Mark, especially where the welfare of clients was concerned.

Ann's insistence on strict standardization prevailed. In fact, it started the process that led to accreditation, which would become a company turning point. Ann says, "We're now known for quality, skilled care."

As Mark had hoped, Ann quickly emerged as a leader. She made waves, but most of her colleagues appreciated

ABOVE: No single department or office was responsible for documentation in the 1970s and 1980s, so materials varied widely. The Weekly Time Slip was one of the few consistent documents.

that. "When Ann came to the company, I saw the level of sophistication in nursing at this organization elevate in front of my eyes. That was a critical point for BAYADA," says Anne Johnson, who joined in 1984 and is the Division Director of Policy Development.

Because Ann was in charge of the form standardization, among many other responsibilities, Mark would often phone her with questions about particular forms. He invited her to meetings about them—meetings that required Ann to travel from Willow Grove to Moorestown. That's a 60-mile roundtrip drive. Before long, Mark was asking her to attend all kinds of meetings. By then, Ann was on to him. "I was always a little suspicious about the meetings that had nothing to do with rehab nursing," she laughs.

"When I started here, I remember saying to my director, 'May I see your policy book?' She said no. I asked, 'Why not?' She said, 'We don't have one.' Soon we did. We became certified. Today BAYADA is a preferred provider for a lot of hospitals and insurance companies because they know the quality of care we give."

ELLEN WIEST, RN, CRRN, who started in 1989 and is a Clinical Manager in Burlington County, New Jersey

LEFT: Upon her hiring in 1989, Ann plunged into the standardization of hundreds of clinical forms and procedures. Her leadership in this area was transformative, because it made processes more efficient and led to the company's first accreditation.

Love in bloom

From their initial meeting onward, Mark and Ann knew they had a lot in common personally and professionally. Given the family atmosphere at BAYADA, they didn't just talk about company matters. They also chatted about their kids, who were close in age. It wasn't long before both of them felt a romantic spark.

Mark had a strict "no dating employees" policy. Under his self-imposed rule, he felt that if he and Ann became a couple, she'd have to leave the company. It was very unlike Mark to go against his own rule, but he and Ann decided that a low-key date couldn't hurt.

BELOW: Mark and Ann's courtship included plenty of family outings with all five kids. This was one of the first. Left to right in 1991: Kelli, Janice, Jackie, David, and Christin.

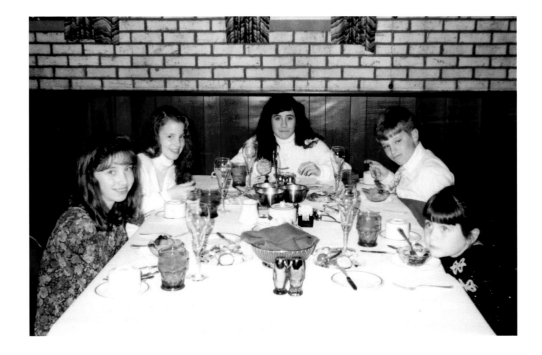

At the same time, they both believed that strong relationships with their kids and between the kids would be essential if they were to have a future together. After a short time dating, they decided to take the five youngsters to a family-friendly restaurant. And it was a success.

"I've always loved Mark," says Kelli, Ann's middle daughter. From that very first gathering, she liked being around him. Looking back, Ann's daughters say that Mark had a comforting effect on all of them. He is a happy dad, with a limitless well of paternal love. "There was space for Mark to fill and we needed it," says Jackie, the oldest daughter. "I wouldn't have identified it as relief at the time, but we were happy about them being together."

The first family date led to several more. "We wouldn't just go out on a Saturday night. We'd plan a whole Saturday with the kids," Ann says.

From preschooler Christin to 12-year-olds Jackie and David, everyone got along. Kelli and Janice bonded almost immediately. "Us" and "them" feelings rarely arose—a remarkable situation that has never changed. Granted, David was the only boy, but the girls teased him that they were preparing him for an all-female future. (They were right, as David grew up to have two daughters.)

The gestation of the new family, and the emotional support it brought, came at a particularly good time. Before Mark and Ann started dating, Mark had lost his father to colon cancer. After Larry's passing, Mark's mom, who had experienced a stroke several years prior, moved in with Mark, David, and Janice. Larry had always insisted on caring for his wife, Anne, by himself. Now Mark hired a BAYADA

Home Health Aide for her. While the aide helped out mainly when David and Janice were at school, they saw enough of her to experience home health care firsthand. This personal exposure at a young age helped both of them to better understand how their family business helped families.

In his energetic yet serene way, Mark kept on top of all his responsibilities. His goals remained consistent: Keep his family happy, his clients happy, and his employees happy; grow the business in a responsible way. But what about his "no dating employees" rule? As their relationship grew serious, Mark and Ann tried to keep it quiet. That lasted about three months. "We did it secretly, which drove me crazy because I don't like to keep secrets," says Mark.

Meanwhile, the rehabilitation nursing business was blossoming. Still, by 1990, it came time to make a decision about Ann's future at the company. Being a sensitive, thoughtful man as well as a devotee of consensus, Mark decided to see what others thought. He called some of the office directors and asked their opinion on Ann staying at BAYADA Nurses.

Ann picks up the story: "Mark said, 'I want to talk to you about something: I'm dating Ann Claffey. And if you have an issue with that, tell me now, because if most people have an issue with that, Ann is prepared to leave.'" They weren't kidding. Mark had promised to help Ann find another job if it came to that.

One of those directors at the time, Carole McMahon, recalls it well. Early on, she says, "I could see that there was some attraction there. When they were dating, Mark asked us how we felt about it. I supported them, because I knew

both of them and I could tell that they were good for each other. Ann's a wonderful person and she shares his vision. They're a perfect couple."

Not only did the overwhelming majority of directors give Mark and Ann their resounding approval, but a few even said their courtship was long overdue.

A festive wedding

The happy couple knew they wanted to marry. In January 1991, Mark proposed and Ann accepted. As their plans progressed, they brought the kids together for family meetings. There, they talked about their feelings and discussed how their households would come together.

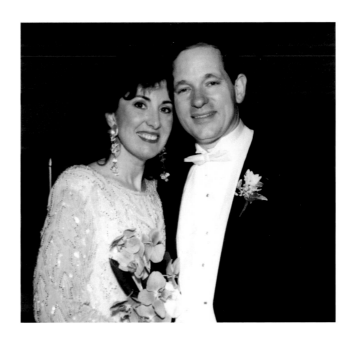

LEFT: The blissful couple at their wedding on July 28, 1991. Both in their early 40s, Mark and Ann felt they had finally found their soulmates.

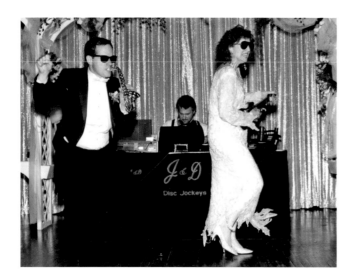

ABOVE: Attended by 476 guests, Mark and Ann's reception served as a wedding celebration, a company party, and a family reunion.

BELOW: Ann's sister Carolyn Meyers, a BAYADA Nurse, posed with their father, James Claffey, for company marketing materials in the 1990s. Their mother, Edith, also appeared in some photos. It was Mark's idea to use them as models, partly because he is famously thrifty, but also as a loving gesture to Ann and his in-laws.

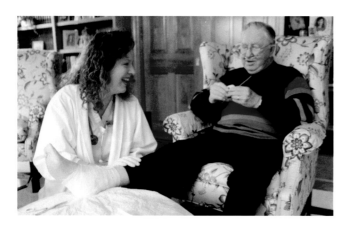

"It was so different from other divorced families who remarry and the kids are the afterthoughts. We were the first priority," says Christin. "It wasn't about just the two of them at all."

Together, they agreed on a wedding date: July 28, 1991. In true Baiada and BAYADA fashion, the wedding was all about family. A total of 476 people were in attendance, mostly Baiada and Claffey family members as well as many in the BAYADA Nurses family. In fact, the event was three-fold: a wedding, a company party, and a family reunion. At the time, BAYADA held quarterly company parties. It so happened the wedding fell at the end of the quarter, so all of the office employees were invited. The annual reunion of the extended Baiada family usually took place at that time of year, too, at the Jersey shore, so Mark's large family was already going to be in town as well.

Much like company parties, the wedding reception was wildly fun and festive. At the introductions, the deejay honored the children in a special way. As he introduced them, a video parody of *The Brady Bunch,* the popular 1970s television series about a blended family, played behind them. Each of the Baiada family members' photos appeared in a different square, just like the opening montage of the TV show. The Baiada Bunch, as they love to refer to themselves, was born.

After the wedding, Mark and Ann headed for their honeymoon in Avalon, New Jersey, where they were joined by 76 family members from both sides. Their "romantic getaway" actually took place at the site of the weekend-long Baiada family reunion. "That was my first clue what my life was going to be like," says Ann with a chuckle.

"I wish everyone could see Mark and Ann together. They're a hoot. They're a couple in love still. I remember one Awards Weekend when he got down on one knee and gave her roses. It was her twentieth year at the company. In every setting Ann just breaks the ice with everyone. They're real. Really real and no pretense, just down-to-earth."

KAREN HOJDA, who joined in 2001 and is Director of Leadership Development and Talent Management, Burlington, New Jersey

"So close to home"

It's never easy to learn that a loved one is dealing with a chronic or catastrophic illness that will require home health care. Throughout BAYADA's history, many of its own employees have felt uniquely comforted to have their family members cared for by fellow employees.

Mark's own mother, Anne, was a BAYADA client for 20 years, and lived with his family the entire time. "My kids and I all experienced home care firsthand," he says. He adds his mom was picky, but lucky to have some aides who became like family members.

When retiree Bonnie Carr Long's mother became ill in 2011, it presented a logistical problem as her mom lived in Maryland and Bonnie was in Pennsylvania. But employees in some Pennsylvania, Delaware, and Maryland offices "went out of their way" to get an available aide from Pennsylvania certified in Maryland, according to Bonnie, who was then the company's Manager of Special Projects. "They even drove the home health aide to Baltimore to obtain the certification in advance," Bonnie recalls with gratitude.

An effective routine began: Bonnie would drive the live-in aide from Pennsylvania on

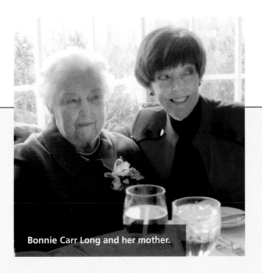

Bonnie Carr Long and her mother.

Wednesdays and pick her up 10 days later for a break. When that aide had to leave after several months for health reasons, colleagues found another compassionate, excellent, and reliable aide for Bonnie's mom. "When you have people who will go to that extent for you, they're really pretty special people, and they make you feel special," says Bonnie. "The BAYADA office employees and field employees made it possible for my mother to live at home, where she wanted to be. She was safe and happy and I felt secure knowing she was in such good care."

Maureen Wright couldn't agree more. In 2000, her brother, who was 43 at the time, experienced a stroke. Doctors advised his family to place him in a nursing home. Having worked as an Area Director for 20 years in Philadelphia, Maureen knew better. He recovered at home, thanks to BAYADA nursing services and the help of Maureen's extended family.

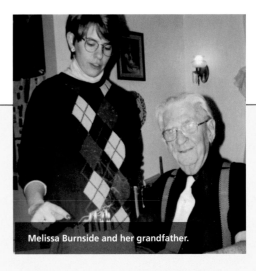

Melissa Burnside and her grandfather.

"It just makes it so personal when you have family members who are being helped by what we do," says Karen Hojda, Director of Leadership Development and Talent Management in Burlington, New Jersey. BAYADA has cared for Karen's grandmother, stepfather, and close neighbors.

Melissa Burnside also knows that feeling. In the early 2000s, Melissa's grandfather, who had cancer, lived with her family. During that time, he required a BAYADA live-in aide as well as visiting home health aides. As Division Director in Parsippany, New Jersey, she knew the great work BAYADA does, but the true extent literally "hit home" then. "It was the most honest thing that my family could have experienced," Melissa says. "I always knew the work we do is meaningful, but when it came to my home, it really gave me a different perspective."

Leading with humility

You might expect the head of one of the nation's leading home health care companies to fit the CEO stereotype: reserved, cautious, focused only on the bottom line. Instead, Mark Baiada is a rock star to those who know him. Mark is fun. Mark is open-minded. Mark is caring. And maybe most importantly, Mark is genuine and down-to-earth.

Admired for his warm, approachable nature as well as his intellect and business savvy, Mark influences people without proselytizing. His personality is pervasive in BAYADA's culture. "I watch how it plays out in other people's decision-making and dialogue, in all kinds of settings and situations," says his son, David Baiada, Chief Operating Officer, Home Health, Hospice, and Quality. "I think it has been the cultural glue throughout our history. People ask themselves, 'What would Mark do in this situation?'"

Janice Lovequist, Mark's daughter and Manager of *The BAYADA Way* Team, still has to urge him to see the power of his involvement in companywide communications. "Sometimes I'm thinking, 'You don't get it. You don't get

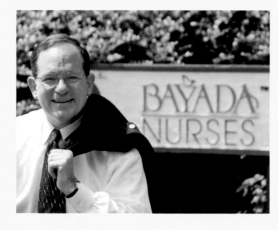

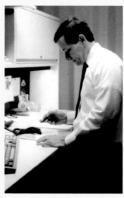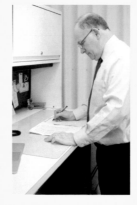

TOP: Mark at Headquarters in 2008.

ABOVE: Mark at his Chester Avenue desk circa 1985 and in 2015. He is comfortable with modest, well-used furniture and equipment, a fact that sometimes frustrates Ann.

how much you're respected, how much more important messages are when they come from you.'"

Daughter Kelli Marans, Compliance Counsel for BAYADA, agrees. "In webinars, even though Mark is talking to thousands of people, people get really excited about seeing him and hearing what he has to say," says Kelli. "He quotes *The BAYADA Way* in every meeting. He can bring everything back to the simple words of *The BAYADA Way* without fail. And I think people just really love it."

Sharon Vogel, Director of Hospice Services, actually envisions a little Mark Baiada on her shoulder to consult in frustrating situations, from traffic jams to business negotiations. "He's really taught me the importance of maintaining perspective, that this is a people business first, and you're always going to be surrounded by difficult situations," says Sharon. "He's shown me how to deal with challenges in a healthy manner and not to lose it."

Despite his strong influence, Mark remains a master of the light touch. Humility counts for a lot with him—he strives for it himself and

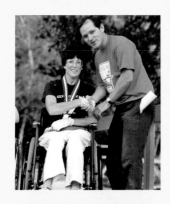

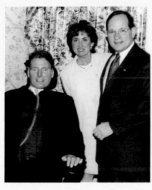

TOP: Mark at the 1987 BAYADA Regatta, congratulating an awardee.

ABOVE: Among the many causes supported by the Baiadas is the Geoffrey Lance Foundation, which hosted an event with actor Christopher Reeve in 2000.

admires it in others. "I don't know that Mark's changed, and that's what makes him so special," says Carole McMahon, Division Director in Haverford, Pennsylvania, who has known him since she joined BAYADA in 1980. "He consistently treats people well, regardless of the circumstance."

Jean Mullin agrees. "Mark shares. It's a fact that he shares the compliments; he shares the money; he shares everything," says Jean, who is Division Director of Adult Nursing and Assistive Care covering Maryland and Delaware, based in Wilmington, Delaware.

Because Mark is genuine, he isn't concerned about putting on airs. For example, his small office at the Moorestown headquarters for some 30 years was hardly what one would expect of a nationwide company president. Its furniture consisted of a metal filing cabinet and a small, round meeting table that doubled as his desk. As Mark's wife, Ann, would often quip: "Every director has a nicer office than Mark's." When BAYADA announced its move to a new headquarters in 2015—a historic home on Main Street in Moorestown, New Jersey, that the

company would renovate— Ann had to insist that Mark occupy one of the bigger spaces.

When it's snowing hard and the roads are hazardous, Mark will walk the mile to work early in the morning rather than risk an accident. It's no surprise that his car is an economical Toyota Prius. Historically, he has also worked late on Christmas Eve and New Year's Eve when others are long gone. Year in and year out, he sets the precedent that guides BAYADA's mission of compassion, excellence, and reliability. 🌿

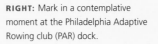

RIGHT: Mark in a contemplative moment at the Philadelphia Adaptive Rowing club (PAR) dock.

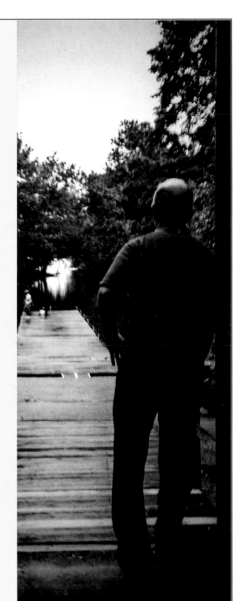

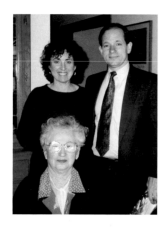

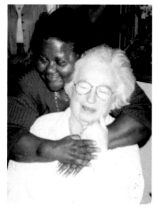

ABOVE: Mark's mom Anne moved into Mark's household after her husband's passing. She continued to live with the family after Mark and Ann's marriage, with help from BAYADA Home Health Aides, including her beloved Connie.

Blending the families

In August 1991, Ann and her girls moved into a new house in Moorestown with the Baiadas. As happy as the blended family was, they all felt some stress. Ann's parents and close friends in Pennsylvania—her long-treasured support system—weren't right around the corner anymore. The girls had to start at a new school. Moorestown Friends School is a congenial place, and David and Janice were very happy there, but still it wasn't easy. Jackie and Kelli were teenagers and had left behind a solid group of established friends. At home, David and Janice weren't used to having a new mother's influence, more people in the house, and new rules to follow. Mark's parental style had been a little more casual than Ann's.

Mark's mom Anne, called Grandmom, still lived with them, too. "It's difficult to have a person with a disability live with you for years and years," her daughter-in-law Ann says. "And home health aides can feel very intrusive to a family. To have a new marriage, raise five kids, and also have a parent with a disability living with us—it was tough. So I thoroughly understand the situation home care families are in."

At the same time, as Ann readily adds, "Grandmom brought love and levity to the family. She was a kind person with a great sense of humor who wouldn't hesitate to laugh at herself. She never wanted to appear a burden." The family included her in every outing. And although she had limited speech, she found ways to tease Mark and offer her opinions. As she tuned into the new dynamics of the household, she would often pipe up with "Mark, Ann is right! Ann is right!"

"I remember thinking, 'Great! Thanks, Mom. Now all the women are ganging up on me,'" Mark says, with affection.

While the blending of the families included a few rough patches, the family got through them with patience and understanding. They became a close, cohesive unit, not least because Mark and Ann insisted on eating a family dinner together every night.

"No matter how much work they had to do and how busy life got, we religiously ate dinner together every single night. I'm not exaggerating. Every single night. When the last person came home, that's when we ate," says Jackie. "Sometimes Mark headed back to work, and Mom did paperwork late into the night, but it was important to them we were together for dinner." The ritual was not lost on the children, who continue it with their own families.

Goals and challenges of the 1990s

The early 1990s brought business transformations as well as personal ones. The company had expanded to 22 service offices and two support offices (accounting and data processing). Although BAYADA hadn't quite reached Hollywood, it had moved well beyond Philadelphia and southern New Jersey to make significant inroads in Wilmington, Delaware; Winston-Salem, North Carolina; and Tampa, Florida—all areas in which its name wasn't known at first.

Ginny Gotides, a retired Division Director who was instrumental in building the Delaware business, describes the typical situation. "In the beginning, we had a meeting with a Wilmington hospital that had its own home care

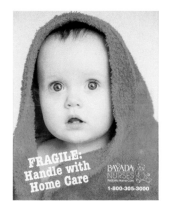

ABOVE: This BAYADA Nurses pediatric ad from the 1990s still brings a smile to employees and clients.

TOP RIGHT: Headquarters employees outside 290 Chester Avenue in Moorestown in 1995.

RIGHT: Offices continually celebrate the company's growth with parties.

BELOW: From the BEARS operating system onward, Mark's love for bears has resonated throughout the company.

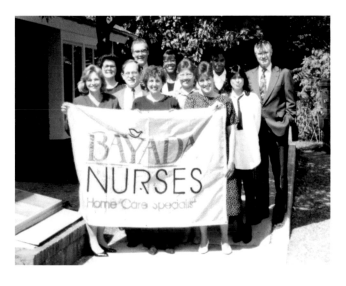

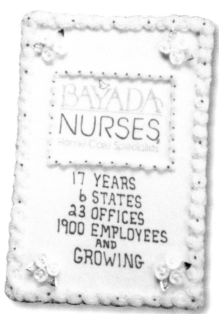

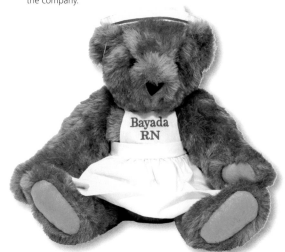

department and visiting nurses. The situation wasn't promising. Mark said we needed to try for three referrals a week," says Ginny. "We laughed about it a lot over the years because three referrals a week quickly turned into a hundred. It's just really a process of growth, forming relationships with the referral sources by providing really good service, and having all your clients who go back to the hospital say, 'I'll have BAYADA Nurses back; they were great.'"

The expansion led to record-breaking weeks in billing. When the company reached an all-time record in October 1991, Mark gratefully said to employees, "It's very exciting to grow. However, as we get larger, I want us all to keep our humble, small company feeling and belief in hard work and basic values. It gives me chills when someone says BAYADA Nurses is 'really good.' Thank you." His caution was astute, because the company had achieved significant momentum. Maintaining that "humble, small company feeling" within a fast-growing organization would become a more pressing challenge.

From the beginning, Mark's values of hard work, honesty, and integrity have guided BAYADA. Employees have taken his lead, and together they've developed the company's outstanding reputation. Maintaining that reputation was most important to Mark as well as to BAYADA's future success. He has never forgotten the words his mother told him as a child, "Reputation is like fine crystal: easy to break and difficult to mend."

Mark knew that a hard-earned reputation can be tarnished in an instant. As an example, he cites the story of an employee's mother experiencing substandard care in a

"Mark always talks about audacious goals. I always did, too. I think that's been part of our success. As a Division Director, I set my goals far into the future. It was fun to do that, to see some people buy into it and grow to become Directors, Area Directors, and Division Directors."

WERNER HOPPE, who joined in 1992 and is a Division Director

Harry, home at last

Harry had never lived on his own. Born with cerebral palsy, he was cared for at home until age 12, when his mother died. By then his condition was too difficult for his father to handle. Because professional home care was not available in the 1940s, Harry's father had no choice but to put him in a nursing home. And there he stayed—until he was 65.

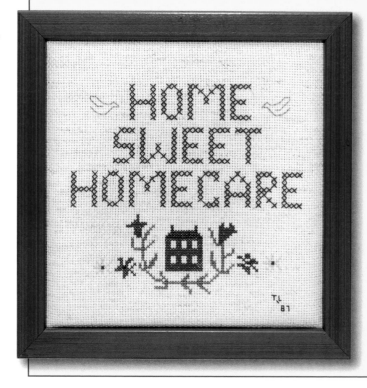

But following a class action lawsuit in the late 1990s, Medicaid clients like Harry finally had the opportunity to receive subsidized care in the community. That enabled BAYADA to move Harry and a few other individuals needing 24-hour-a-day care into the same apartment building (a "client cluster"), where BAYADA Home Health Aides provided care.

It was a new beginning for all concerned. Previously institutionalized clients could now turn to companies such as BAYADA, and those companies could afford to care for them. For Harry, the legal decision also opened the door to a world of personal decisions. For instance, when aides let him pick out what to wear, he had trouble deciding—he'd never had the choice at the nursing home. When asked what he wanted to eat, Harry was equally stumped—he'd never had the freedom to choose. But confronting indecision proved to be a good problem, and Harry lived happily in his new apartment home until he passed away at age 72.

"Our aides became Harry's family and provided a quality of life he never would have known otherwise," says Maureen Wright, Area Director of Philadelphia Specialized Contracts. "To me, that represents why we do what we do." 🌿

LEFT: A sampler cross-stitched for Mark by employee Terri Lupinetti in 1987.

nursing home. "She visited her mother one day and was just so upset that the caregivers allowed her mom to sit there with her sweater on backwards," says Mark. "It's like that one moment when you can feel everything at once—how important the work we do is, every detail, down to keeping people's sweaters on the right way."

Accreditation and other pivotal steps

Having developed a solid reputation and standardized its business processes, BAYADA was ready for the next major step: accreditation by the Joint Commission on the Accreditation of Healthcare Organizations (JCAHO). The process began in 1991, and it required the company to articulate in writing all of its operational policies and practices, which numbered more than 1,000. Since some of the policies were being fully documented for the first time, the work was painstaking. Day by day, month by month, the work progressed. The company earned its first JCAHO accreditation in 1993.

"It was a very proud moment," confirms Marie Blessington, RN, Director of Clinical Leadership Development, who joined the company in 1985. "We went from being a 'handshake company' to one that had rules and regulations and policies. It verified to the world what we already knew, that we really do home care well."

Accreditation came during a pivotal decade for U.S. health care. With costs rising at double the rate of inflation, the cost-cutting mechanism of managed care took hold in the 1990s. The rise of HMOs and the ascendancy of insurers as decision-makers caused confusion for health care

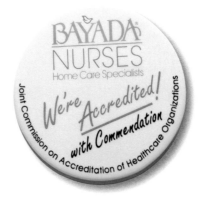

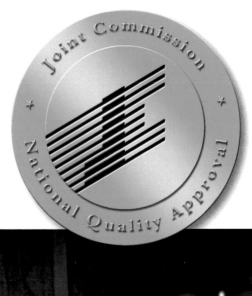

ABOVE: JCAHO accreditation raised the company to a new level.

BELOW: Mark, Sherri Pillet, and Laurel Trice shepherded the rigorous, two-year accreditation process. The company honored Sherri and Laurel's hard work at a 1994 party.

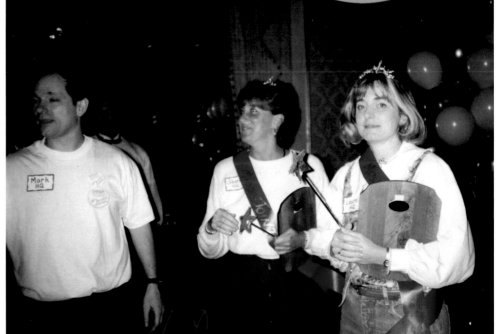

providers, administrators, and especially, clients. Mark and Linda Siessel, who would go on to become the company's Chief Operating Officer, Home Care Services, decided that BAYADA needed a centralized system to deal with the many nuances and challenges of managed care. So in 1995, it opened an office dedicated to handling the managed care learning curve and charged it with the massive task of building bridges with the insurance companies.

"I feel rewarded in that we solve problems when we work with these insurance companies. It's our focus. We get

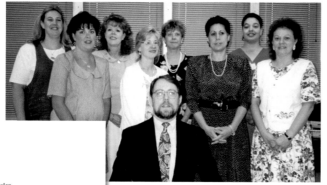

to know them," says Melissa Burnside, Division Director of the Managed Care Office, who started the office and has led it since. "We make relationships and impressions on them so that our offices and our clients can have a positive experience—so they don't have to worry about all those behind-the-scenes details." Reflecting the paradigm shift in health care, the Managed Care Office has grown from a staff of two—Melissa and a nurse—to some 120 people in three locations.

Similarly, exciting growth was happening elsewhere. One example: Maureen Hixon, now Regional Director in Hyannis, Massachusetts, recalls getting a call from a headhunter for BAYADA in 1997. She had just taken a job with another home health care company in order to return to her native New England. Having worked in Pennsylvania previously, however, she knew of and admired BAYADA. One step led to another, and soon she was talking with Linda Siessel and Mark. "After interviewing me for two hours by phone, Mark said, 'How about opening an office on Cape Cod?' Not really knowing him yet, I thought, 'He must be crazy. Open an office? Nobody here knows who BAYADA Nurses is.' But from the moment I talked with Linda and Mark, the philosophy behind this entire company resonated with me. If I could have opened my own home care agency, BAYADA is what I would have created."

BAYADA started in Hyannis in 1997 from a desk in Maureen's dining room. The operation moved into an office in January of 1998 and grew steadily. "We split Hyannis and opened an office in Falmouth. I became an Area Director and then opened up another office. Once you open up so

"Hope lives here"

Seeing a driver in need, Antonio pulled over to the side of the road to help. Unfortunately, this off-duty firefighter's kind deed caused a passing motorist to hit him. The force of the impact resulted in broken bones, massive internal injuries, and traumatic brain injury for Antonio. His chances for survival and recovery were slim.

Despite the odds, Antonio survived. "He is a fighter," says Marie Blessington, RN, Director of Clinical Leadership Development.

After months of acute care and rehabilitation, Antonio was discharged to his home in Quincy, Massachusetts. There, another agency cared for him, but didn't meet his rehabilitation potential. His health, mobility, and optimism diminished.

Then BAYADA got involved and the situation turned around. Through an aggressive rehabilitation plan led by the BAYADAbility team, Antonio was able to stand after a few months. Eventually, he walked. He has returned to a full, rich life, requiring minimal care and attending only outpatient rehab.

"Antonio recovered beyond everyone's expectations," says Marie. "When I was leaving his home after a visit, I noticed a welcome sign. I remember thinking that a more appropriate sign would be one that simply stated, 'Hope lives here!'"

many offices, you move into a Division Director role. Within our region, we have six different divisions now. We've developed Massachusetts and Vermont and are moving into New Hampshire," Maureen says. This pattern continued in other regions. Another contributor to growth, Maureen believes, is the company's track record for employee longevity. "Many people in health care change positions every five years or so, because if you want to move ahead, that's what you need to do. BAYADA is different. What keeps people here? The culture and the opportunity for growth."

BELOW: These custom-made Mark Baiada nesting dolls display name tags that illustrate the career progression that's possible at BAYADA. This idea was originally conceived by Regional Director Melinda Phillips, Director of Hospice Services Sharon Vogel, and Division Director Virginia Steelman to be used as an educational tool in the office employee on-boarding process.

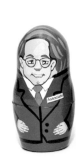
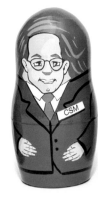
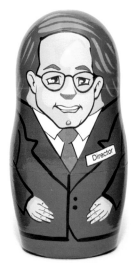
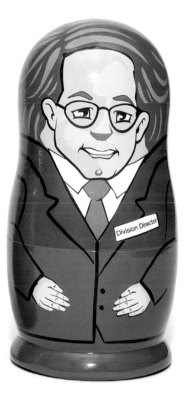

An angel answers a callout plea

While working as a new Staff Supervisor (now called Client Services Manager) in Winston-Salem, North Carolina, Melinda Phillips sometimes felt discouraged. She had moved up to the role from Assistant Home Care Coordinator (similar to today's Associate role), so she figured she was doing something right. At the same time, Melinda found the work stressful and wondered "whether I'd stick it out for even a year."

One morning, Melinda took a call from a woman who said she hadn't slept for days. She had been caring for her sister around the clock and was "desperate for help." Melinda stopped thinking about her own feelings and focused on the woman's needs. "I really connected with her. I remember thinking that I've got to help this lady," she says. She urged the woman not to worry, assuring her that help was on the way.

But several field employees had already "called out" that day, leaving Melinda with no caregivers to call on. "The office staff thought I was crazy for saying I would try to get someone out there," she says. Melinda started to feel as desperate as the caller. Instinctively, she rested her head on her desk and appealed to a higher power: "God, if you really want me to help this lady

and there's someone out there, you're going to have to send them, because I have no idea."

Minutes later, the office doorbell rang. In walked Jackie R., one of the office's best home health aides, who had been out of state visiting family for a few months. The way Melinda greeted her certainly surprised her: "Jackie! I think you're an angel!"

Jackie responded, "Well, I'm not sure about that. But it's the weirdest thing, Melinda. I was in the grocery store and something told me to come over here. So I came."

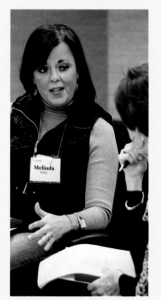

Melinda called the client's sister back, and Jackie headed straight to the client's home. From that moment on, Melinda knew she'd make it in the job and stay in the field because she believed she was part of something greater than herself. Twenty years after starting with BAYADA in 1994, Melinda is now a Regional Director. 🌿

RIGHT: Regional Director Melinda Phillips in 2014 at *The BAYADA Way* retreat in North Carolina.

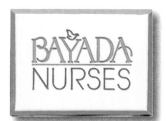

ABOVE: This pin was the result of hands-on engineering by Mark. Dissatisfied with the quality of pins by a vendor, he bought a machine and hand-made the pins and name tags himself. Starting with plastic pins, Mark stacked two layers. Then he engraved a portion of the pin, applied red paint, and wiped away the excess. When it dried, he engraved the second portion deep enough to expose the gray bottom layer.

Benefits of BAYADAbility

Ann Baiada worked diligently toward the goal she and Mark had agreed on when he hired her in 1989: to continue to raise the bar in home care excellence by establishing a more formalized rehabilitation nursing program. Gradually and solidly, Ann built the foundation over the course of a decade. Ann and the company put appropriate policies in place, hired more Certified Rehabilitation Registered Nurses (CRRNs), and gained a reputation as an emerging leader for this specialty in the home care setting. The BAYADAbility program officially launched in 1998. The timing was fortuitous, as client demand was growing.

For clients with severely limited function resulting from catastrophic injury or illness the prospect of being discharged home brings relief—and anxiety. New challenges can await them at home: a home setting that's difficult to navigate as well as being dependent on others for care. The BAYADAbility program works to streamline care for BAYADA's most complex clients.

As a consultative service, BAYADAbility CRRNs help support Clinical Managers after clients' needs have been identified. Together, they work to develop a solution. For example, prior to a client's discharge, a BAYADAbility Nurse can meet with the client and family in the hospital to assess the diagnosis and work with the Clinical Manager to devise a care plan. Working closely with doctors, therapists, insurance companies, and equipment providers, the CRRN also makes recommendations about care and equipment. He or she may visit the client's home to assess the adaptability of the environment, equipment needs, safety, and accessibility.

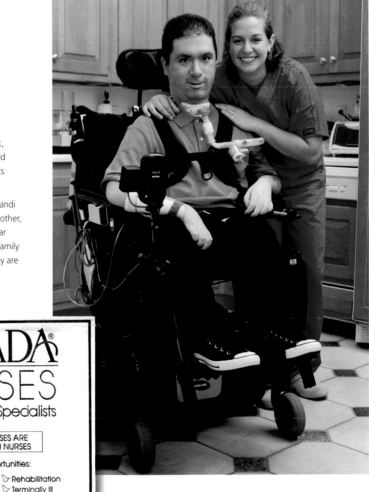

BELOW: Thanks to Ann's work, BAYADA Nurses was able to add rehabilitation as a specialty in its ads and marketing materials.

RIGHT: Client Adam B. and Brandi Lapadula, RN. Adam and his brother, Denny, have Duchenne muscular dystrophy. With support from family and BAYADA professionals, they are living a full life.

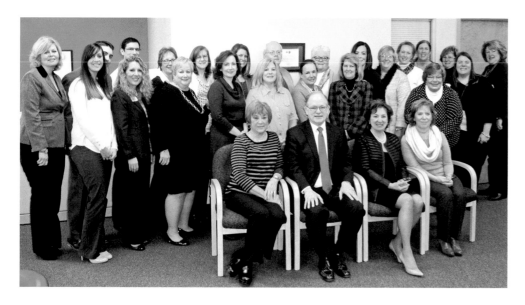

ABOVE: The BAYADAbility clinical team members at the New Jersey Learning Center in 2015. Ann presented the group with an award from the Association of Rehabilitation Nurses (ARN).

BACK ROW: Pamela Soni, Wesley Trice, Anthony D'Alonzo, Jane Feldman, Teresa Lee, Beth Taylor, Charles Veal, LuAnn Trout, Karen Troy, Marilyn Newton, Lisa Fiore, Betsy Bates, Carol Bishop, Cristin Toscano, Mary Ellen Garofalo

MIDDLE ROW: Jessica Rosofsky, Stacey Rice, Carole McMahon, Rosemary Beaumont, Andrea Lavoie, Carmella Love, Maureen Baker, Cay Ambrose

SEATED: Ellen Wiest, Mark Baiada, Ann Baiada, Sharon Driscoll

BELOW: Team members lovingly presented this gavel to their leader Ann, who likes meetings to be orderly.

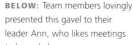

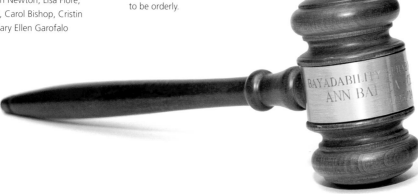

The CRRN will then support the office, client, and family during the transition home.

Clients benefiting from the program include those with spinal cord injury, traumatic brain injury, multiple sclerosis, amyotrophic lateral sclerosis (ALS), muscular dystrophy, cerebral palsy, orthopedic conditions, amputations, and congenital abnormalities as well as those with various catastrophic illnesses and injuries. BAYADAbility can also benefit pediatric clients who require changes to their care plan and equipment due to their growth and development.

As the company has grown, technological advances have allowed BAYADAbility Nurses to reach far and wide. With mobile devices and video conferencing, CRRNs are now able to support and consult remotely in areas that do not have a dedicated rehab nurse—thus helping even more clients navigate that complex passage between hospital and home, ensuring a home life with comfort, independence, and dignity.

Nurse Lisa and "the commercial"

The late 1990s also brought a dramatic surge in the public visibility of BAYADA Nurses. The company produced its first television commercial, an ad so effective that many viewers still remember it vividly. Some even think it's still running. It's a wordless drama called "Heroes on the Home Front," a phrase that BAYADA trademarked.

The commercial, also known as "The Storm," opens with a dark and stormy night. A nameless nurse gets drenched entering her car, grabs her phone once inside, and tells the caller she's on her way. (Keep in mind that mobile phones were a rarity in the 1990s.) Driving white-knuckled through the storm with sirens sounding in the background, she stops to check her map to find a better route. Soon she arrives, beeping the horn to greet her client, a man with quadriplegia. His ventilator is visible as he waits for her by the front window. Upon her arrival, he manages a smile of relief. Cut!

In the voiceover to this dramatic 30-second spot, the narrator says, "BAYADA Nurses. Their tradition was forged on the battlefield. Today, they serve on a field just as challenging: The home front. Where often getting the call means going beyond the call. BAYADA Nurses: Not everyone can follow in tradition's footsteps, but those who do are truly heroes to those they care for. BAYADA Nurses: Truly Heroes on the Home Front."

"Heroes on the Home Front" debuted on October 4, 1998, in the Philadelphia and Tucson, Arizona, markets. It didn't quite meet its primary purpose as a recruitment tool, as Mark admits: "We kept close track before and after the launch, and there was only a small improvement." However, the emotionally gripping ad catapulted BAYADA into the consciousness of everyone who saw it—so much so that the company ran it for a decade. "The real effect of the 10-year run was awareness, which probably helped recruiting."

The ad was equally memorable for those behind the scenes. Mark couldn't attend the filming, so he volunteered Ann as head technical advisor. She traveled to the location—an abandoned mental hospital in Newtown, Connecticut—with fellow nurse Clare Gallagher and National Accounts Manager Howard Algeo. "We were there to help the nurse look like a nurse, and the client look like a client," Ann recalls. "We had all these different hats,

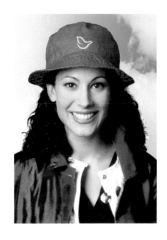

CLOCKWISE: Actress and model Lisa Gorlitsky portrayed Nurse Lisa. She was chosen, in part, for her resemblance to Julianna Margulies, who played a nurse on the TV show *ER*.

The TV commercial presented a gripping drama in just 30 seconds.

Nurse Lisa appeared on refrigerator magnets, BAYADA Bucks, brochures, educational materials, and other printed matter.

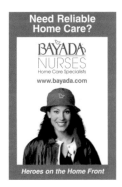

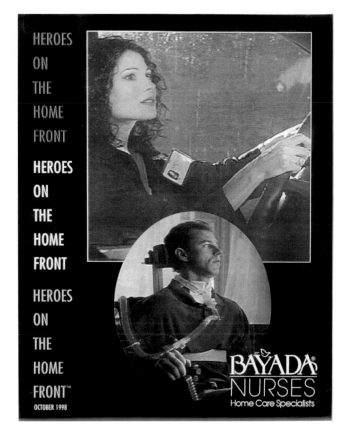

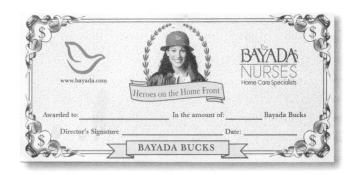

raincoats, and nursing pins. The nurse wears my mother's nursing pin in the commercial."

Created by a New Jersey ad agency and produced for a thrifty $200,000, the commercial involved a director, a 50-person crew, and catered meals. "I felt like I was with Steven Spielberg on a movie set," Ann recalls. "It was so much fun!" The crew filmed over two nights from 6:00 P.M. to 6:00 A.M. Setting the commercial in the dark of night, says Ann, "made it scarier and more important for the nurse to get there."

As for the storm, it was generated by a towering machine attached to a fire hydrant. Ann recalls that "the director would say, 'Give me rain!' and it would pour from this machine, which was higher than a big tree. Nurse Lisa was constantly getting soaked." The character was played by actress and model Lisa Gorlitsky, who had been chosen for her resemblance to actress Julianna Margulies, then popular for her portrayal of hard-working nurse Carol Hathaway in the TV show *ER*.

Nurse Lisa, as BAYADA dubbed her, became the company's public face. For years, she appeared on recruitment posters, brochures, and even a huge billboard in downtown Philadelphia.

"Every time you would see that commercial, you would be proud of it," says Marty (Martha) Soroka, Division Director of the Personal Care Assistant office in Philadelphia, who has been with BAYADA since 1977. "It made such a difference. People really did recognize the BAYADA name. Our aides even mentioned how proud they were." The commercial can still be seen on YouTube, where it has been viewed more than 10,000 times.

RIGHT: Mark and Ann present a 2011 National Hero Award to Barbara Sauer, a Medical Social Worker in the home health service office in Denver, Colorado. All National Heroes of the Year from 2000 onward are listed in an appendix to this book.

BELOW: A button made by a service office circa 1997, given for recognition and appreciation of hard work.

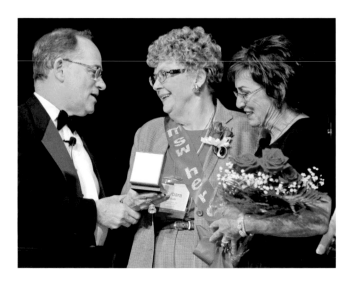

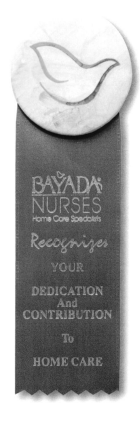

The Hero Program

While the television commercial boosted brand awareness, its strongest legacy is perhaps the Hero on the Home Front Program. The company launched it in 1998 to celebrate its real home care heroes. (The name has since been shortened to the Hero Program.) The linchpin of the company's employee recognition efforts, the program honors RNs, LPNs, home health aides, therapists, and medical social workers who perform beyond expectations. Office employees and clients nominate these individuals, using the three core values of *The BAYADA Way* as criteria: compassion, excellence, and reliability.

Each hero enjoys a recognition party in his or her honor with family members and sometimes even clients in attendance. These heroes are first nominated and honored quarterly with recognition parties at the local office level,

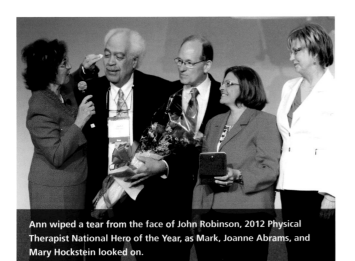

Ann wiped a tear from the face of John Robinson, 2012 Physical Therapist National Hero of the Year, as Mark, Joanne Abrams, and Mary Hockstein looked on.

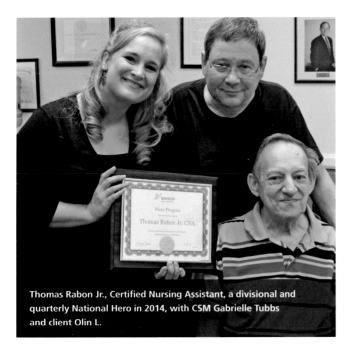

Thomas Rabon Jr., Certified Nursing Assistant, a divisional and quarterly National Hero in 2014, with CSM Gabrielle Tubbs and client Olin L.

"Ready to battle the next thing"

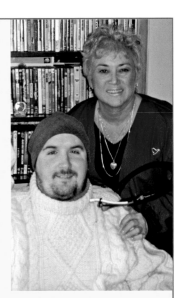

After a motorcycle accident at age 24, Tony L. has lived with quadriplegia for 17 years. The condition hasn't stopped him or diminished his gratitude for his remaining abilities. In the course of a conversation with Ellen Wiest, RN, CRRN, the Clinical Manager who has long overseen his case, Tony casually recalls coming home after one of many complications, "ready to battle the next thing."

"You hear that?" asks Ellen, whose respect for him is evident. "Ready to battle the next thing! His attitude is the best."

Tony uses a sip-and-puff motorized wheelchair that he operates by blowing into a straw. This ingenious device takes him wherever he wants to go both inside and, within limits, outside. In his house, he can control the television, air conditioning, heat, and lights—even the light on his fish tank—and access the internet, all through a computer that uses voice recognition technology. He drives a van adapted for his use by Miles Technologies, funded by A Step Toward Hope and the Christopher Reeve Foundation.

While Tony appreciates the technology that gives him so much independence, he especially cherishes his BAYADA caregivers. "When I first came home from the rehabilitation hospital in 1997, I had aides but couldn't find one that my family and I liked," he recalls. Soon after, he needed a tracheostomy and required more care than before. At that point, he switched to BAYADA. "Once BAYADA started helping me, everything was better. We just stayed with them. We've never had a problem."

ABOVE: Client Tony L. and Ellen Wiest share a long relationship filled with mutual respect.

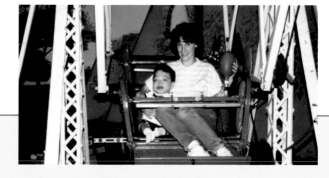

TOP: Joey and his Registered Nurse Donna W., just before they soared into the sky. Donna held the "bagging" equipment that made Joey's Ferris wheel adventure possible. (Bagging is shorthand for squeezing a self-inflating bag to provide ventilation to people who are not breathing or not breathing adequately.) Joey has since passed away, but his mom keeps in touch with BAYADA, and Donna is still with the Pediatric Cherry Hill (New Jersey) office.

BELOW: Portia in the 1990s, with her irresistible smile captured in a snapshot by Marion Fiero. Portia has since passed away.

Like other kids

Pediatric clients have an especially strong grip on BAYADA heartstrings. Their stories could fill an entire book! These two are among the most memorable.

Portia rides a bike

Portia faced immense challenges. But despite using a ventilator and suffering from significant multiple health problems, she wanted to be like other kids. "Portia had a huge personality and a lot of courage," remembers Marion Fiero, Division Director of Home Health in Philadelphia, who's been with BAYADA since 1979. A true "girly girl," Portia loved having nurses braid her hair and paint her nails. Often she demanded it, but always with a cheerful grin. Finding her hard to resist, nurses typically gave in.

One day, Portia wanted to ride a bike—definitely not an easy request to fill for a child who uses a ventilator. But her nurse said she'd find a way. And she did. In the form of training wheels and 100 feet of medical tubing! "The nurse said, 'Okay, you can only go as far as this roll of tubing will go.' She then ran breathlessly behind Portia, letting out the tubing as Portia pedaled along," Marion explains. "This little girl was the best. Oh, she just loved being able to ride a bike and experience what other children do."

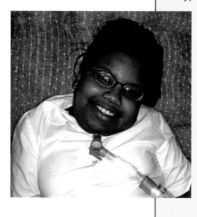

Joey in the sky with BAYADA

Susan (Susie) Ecker Sterner, CSN, BA, loved Joey, a boy with dwarfism who had restrictive lung disease. She started caring for him when he was six and found him to be one of the sweetest clients she'd ever met.

In the 1990s, kids with his condition were typically homebound—their electronic equipment kept them inside. Portable ventilators weren't available yet. But Joey's mother wanted him to have the best possible quality of life, so she and Susie took turns hand-ventilating or "bagging" him in public, including at school.

"When he first started going to school, it was only one class for an hour, just so he could socialize and meet the children. He loved it," says Susie, who joined BAYADA in 1991 and is now a Senior Transitional Care Manager. Her job is to transition patients home from Children's Hospital of Philadelphia, one of the world's most renowned pediatric facilities.

Joey's sense of exploration knew no bounds. When a carnival came to town, he wanted to ride the Ferris wheel! Susie felt some trepidation—the boy's life would be in BAYADA's hands,100 feet above the ground. But with emergency equipment at hand, Joey's nurse and his mom gave him the experience he craved. "We bagged him the whole time," Susie says. "He did great." 🌿

one way that BAYADA nurtures a "small company" feeling as it grows. The Hero Program Committee members then vote on divisional and quarterly national heroes. Finally, four national heroes are chosen and appear on stage at the annual Awards Weekend with their families, where they are applauded by nearly 3,000 BAYADA colleagues.

These amazing winners are honored with documentary videos that draw standing ovations at the annual Awards Weekend celebration. (The heroes' families also attend as all-expense-paid guests of BAYADA and stand on stage with the awardee during the presentation.) The videos remain on the company's YouTube channel as public testimonies to the Heroes.

"The Hero Program awards are always memorable be-cause it drives it home for all of us why we're here. We have thousands of clinicians providing care every day and we're only highlighting a few," says Barbara Colin, MSN, RN, Chief Nursing Officer in Moorestown, New Jersey. "The hero stories are just so representative of the work we do and the dedication. You come away every time crying your eyes out. It's inspiring, and I just love it."

Kosovo and care without boundaries

Since 1975, BAYADA Nurses have excelled at answering the call to local clients in their own homes. In 1999, company nurses began to take that call to an international volunteer level.

Knowing the situation was bleak for refugees of the Kosovo War, Mark spearheaded a volunteer nurse effort to help ease the suffering. The company teamed up with the

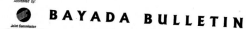
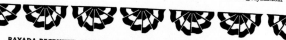

BAYADA BULLETIN

VOL. XIII-NO. 22 June 4, 1999   http://www.bayada.com   e-mail: info@bayada.com

BAYADA RECRUITED 10 VOLUNTEER NURSES FOR RELIEF EFFORT

• Written by **Cheryl Kendra**, Program Development Assistant, CCP

Bayada Nurses has selected its team of ten volunteer nurses to travel to the Balkans and provide relief to the Kosovar refugees. Three of the ten nurses are presently employed by Bayada. One works as a Nursing Supervisor for WIN, the second is a field nurse for AC, and the third is a field nurse for DEN. The others are all concerned residents of the Delaware Valley who responded to Bayada's KYW news radio advertisement.

Eight of ten volunteer applications submitted to the International Medical Corps have already been approved. The nurses' destinations and dates of departure/return have been confirmed by the IMC, as well. The two remaining applications, submitted to the IMC this past week, are currently being processed.

The team of RNs recruited by Bayada Nurses will be traveling either to Skopje, Macedonia or to one of two cities in Albania (Tirana or Kukes), where the IMC has concentrated its relief efforts. They will be working out of tent clinics at the primary boarders or in mobile clinics along the frontier. The first of the volunteers will be dispatched in just a few weeks, leaving 06/20/99 and the last of the approved volunteers will be returning the end of September.

The International Medical Corps revealed that it will be scheduling volunteers to provide relief in the Balkans at least through December. At any given time, it has a rotation of ten volunteers in Macedonia, and a rotation of 12-13 volunteers in Albania. In response to this need, Bayada will determine if any of the remaining applicants who have submitted resumes are interested in a six week minimum volunteer term. If so, travel, room, and board would be provided by the IMC for those qualified.

nonprofit International Medical Corps (IMC), which sends medical personnel to assist relief efforts. The IMC required that nurses could cope with a heavy physical and emotion-al toll. BAYADA took applications and conducted IMC's required background checks. Ultimately, the company sponsored 10 RNs to spend four weeks in the Balkans, caring for injured refugees.

The international stage was set. Eleven years later, BAYADA Nurses responded unstintingly when a catastrophic earthquake hit Haiti. Four nurses volunteered there with IMC and 25 volunteered through Heart to Heart Inter-national for four weeks at a time. The program lasted for more than two years. Four nurses returned for a second stint, one nurse for a third, and one for a fourth. In all, BAYADA

ABOVE: This 1999 *BAYADA Bulletin* article reported on the enthusiastic response to the call for volunteers.

LEFT: A volunteer nurse in the Stenkovec refugee camp. According to the *Croatian Medical Journal,* the "refugee crisis in Macedonia in 1999 was unique in terms of its unprecedented magnitude . . . . Within nine weeks, the country received 344,500 refugees."

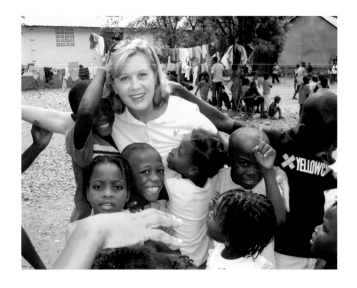

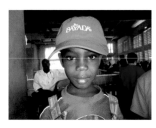

ABOVE AND LEFT: Haitian children helped by Marian B. and other BAYADA Registered Nurse volunteers, who provided more than 1,000 days of coverage in Haiti starting in 2010.

BELOW: Mark impersonated Santa not just on calls to young Wes Trice (shown with his mom, Laurel), but in company skits.

Nurses provided more than 1,000 days of coverage. They shared their experiences and photos with colleagues via a special portal on the company website.

Volunteering for long periods can be financially tough. To ease the burden, BAYADA colleagues pitched in. "People from across the company donated vacation days into a bank that we used for the nurses. And many donated money to a fund to cover the nurses' time," says Bonnie Carr Long, retired Manager of Special Projects. "So there were lots of ways for all employees to participate by assuring financial support to these selfless volunteers. These were heartwarming, satisfying campaigns."

Mark as "Phone Santa"

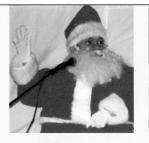

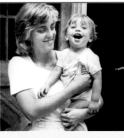

One particular memory from the 1990s still resonates with Laurel Trice and her son, Wesley, who was a preschooler then. As Christmas approached, Laurel casually mentioned to Mark that Wesley was starting to question the idea of Santa Claus. How could Santa know what Wesley wanted for Christmas? And how could the elves make all those toys?

"So Mark came up with the idea of leaving a message on our answering machine at home, while Wes was at day care," recalls Laurel, who is an RN and Director of Clinical Operations of Adult Assistive Care in Burlington, New Jersey. "Every day when we got home, Wes would run to the phone and hit the button for messages and we'd listen to them together. On that day, Wes hit the button and heard 'Ho, ho, ho! Merry Christmas, Wes! I heard that you want new GI Joes and Transformers for Christmas. Well, my elves are working on that right now and they will be there for you on Christmas morning!' If you could have seen the look on my son's face to hear Santa!"

Laurel adds that the story simply illustrates how Mark has an immense effect on people, both big and small. Better yet, she notes that Wesley grew up to work for BAYADA. An early graduate of the company's Associate Leadership Development Program, he started an office in Boston, left to earn his MBA degree, and returned to work as a Director with Mark on new initiatives. 🌿

Looking ahead

The 1990s had brought major transformations to BAYADA and the Baiada family. The company was about to turn 25. Approaching that milestone prompted Mark to do some extra soul-searching, an activity that is second nature to him. What would the twenty-first century BAYADA look and feel like?

As he had predicted, keeping the tight-knit family feel was a constant challenge. For many years, for example, he had recognized each employee's birthday with a personal phone call. Every December, he would carve out time to call every office and wish each employee the happiest of holidays. But because of BAYADA's phenomenal growth, there were no longer enough hours in the day for Mark to do that—at least for much longer.

Thoughtfulness was a vital part of the culture. Mark embraces technology rather than fears it, and he figured that the growth of computers and the internet could only help in that regard. Every gesture counts: The *BAYADA Bulletin* lists employee birthdays every month, for example, and if Mark couldn't write individual cards, he could compose companywide cards and emails for National Nurses Week, Thanksgiving, and the December holidays. Extra-special holiday gifts could go out to every office employee.

With those thoughts in mind, Mark turned his attention toward the year 2000 and a new chapter in the company's history.

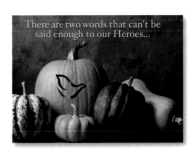

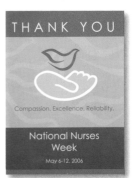

LEFT: A sampling of holiday, Thanksgiving, and National Nurses Week cards that are designed in house and sent to employees annually.

RIGHT: An imaginative employee created this Monopoly®-style home health care game as a gift to the Baiadas. The playing pieces included a nurse's cap, a stethoscope, a telephone, a client using a walker, and a BAYADA dove. The rule sheet said, in part, that "BAYADA Nurses' goals are to play as hard as they work" and "to be recognized and respected for the important games they play."

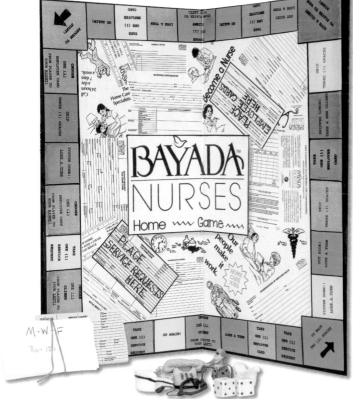

A Conversation with The Baiada Bunch

At the fortieth anniversary of BAYADA Home Health Care, one year shy of Mark and Ann's silver wedding anniversary, the Baiada family includes five children, five spouses, and nine young grandchildren on whom Mark and Ann dote. All of them live in the Philadelphia area, mostly in southern New Jersey.

• **Jaclyn (Jackie) Kirchhoff,** BSN, MSN, has worked in BAYADA's Clinical Standards and Quality (CSQ) office. Jackie and her husband, Michael Kirchhoff, have three children: Katie, age 8; Molly, 6; and Joey, 4.

• **David Baiada** is the company's Chief Operating Officer, Home Health, Hospice, and Quality. David and his wife, Mindy, have two children: Gweneth, age 3, and Annabelle, 2.

• **Kelli Marans,** an attorney, is Compliance Counsel for BAYADA. Kelli and her husband, Jon Marans, have two children: Benjamin, age 3, and Annie, 1.

• **Janice Lovequist** is Manager of *The BAYADA Way* Team. Janice and her husband, Brian Lovequist, have two children: Madelyn, age 5, and William, 3.

• **Christin Gregory** is a Consultant for the company's Hospice Practice. Christin and her husband, David Gregory, are expecting their first child in September 2015.

In December 2014, The Baiada Bunch gathered for a spirited discussion. Here are excerpts.

Mark and Ann, what was it about the other that you fell in love with?

Mark: Ann's personality. She's vivacious and funny. Also, her family orientation, her devotion to home nursing, and her competence at it. And she's a good mom.

Ann: Mark's goodness. His authentic goodness.

Mark: I thought you were going to say it was my good looks.

Baiada children, what can you say about Mark and Ann as a couple?

Christin: They're two very amazing role models.

Kelli: Any time they hear their wedding song, "Unforgettable," they dance in the middle of a restaurant or anywhere else when nobody else is dancing.

Ann: I think we've embarrassed them multiple times.

Kelli: It was an embarrassment when we were young. Now I think it's pride.

Mark: Now we're just a cute older couple.

Jackie: Yeah, when we were teenagers we'd say, "Ah, stop dancing! Nobody else is dancing." Now it's like they're role models for a good marriage.

During your courtship, you began having family meetings. What were some of the most interesting conversations?

Janice: We had a meeting to decide if Pop and Ann should have a child together.

Kelli: It was a unanimous "No!"

Mark: That was my point. This is really pretty good. Everybody's getting along. Why throw something, another person, in the mix? Plus, Christin won't like it.

Christin: Yeah, I'm the baby.

Mark: She was going to lose her special place. I was for you, Chrissy.

Ann: We always made sure all the kids were treated equally. If there was a rule for one, it was for all. If somebody had to do a chore, they all did. There was a rotating chore list on the calendar. They didn't like it always, but it was just the way it was. Nobody got off without doing anything. There was no favoritism. And if we spent this amount on a birthday gift, that's what we spent on the next four kids, too.

What does "family first" mean to you?

Mark: For me, it's just the most important thing. You take care of the family first. Both Ann and I were always taking care of people in need in our homes—my mom, my first wife's brother. If people are in need, you try to help them.

Ann: The idea of taking care of others was really ingrained in both of us. And with our kids.

Jackie: Being home for dinner—that's the example that I will use. Once Mark and my mom got married, that's really when the company started to grow exponentially. But no matter what, we ate dinner together every night.

David: I think it means to make time for dinner and breakfast. It means don't skirt your professional responsibilities, but your primary responsibility is to your family. Take care of your family.

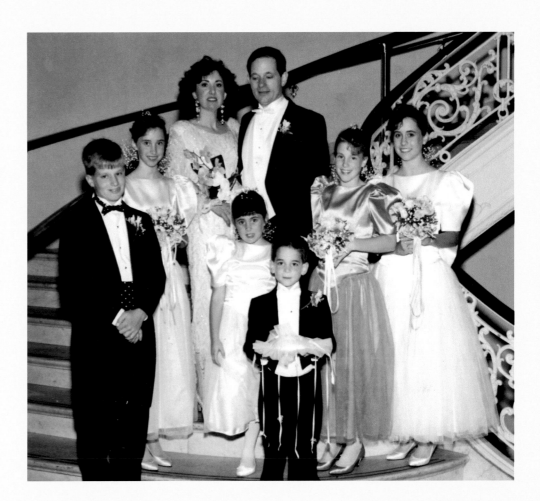

ABOVE: Ann and Mark at their wedding reception on July 28, 1991, with children David, Kelli, Christin, Janice, and Jackie. The ring bearer was Brian Baiada, the son of Mark's brother Matt.

A Conversation with The Baiada Bunch *continued*

Christin: It's an old-school philosophy: You stick together, take care of each other, and spend a lot of time together. Maybe it doesn't happen as much nowadays, but we still maintain that culture as much as we can—with aunts, uncles, and cousins, too.

Kelli: It means that supporting a connected and happy family is our top priority. It's always a balance where there is such important work to be done here or in any other profession, but a strong family provides a good base to do a lot of good in other arenas.

Janice: The whole "family first" idea includes employees, too. It's always been clear that Pop puts both his personal family and his work family above everything else, and he allows his employees to do the same. "Family first" is like an unwritten rule at BAYADA. It's about compassion for others, and it's yet another uniquely amazing thing about the culture Pop has built, both in our family and at BAYADA.

What was it like growing up in a home health care family business?

David: BAYADA was really a community of people, in the early years especially. They spent a lot of time together in the office, at events, at the Regatta. I didn't really understand the business until I got much older, but I remember the people who were good to me.

Janice: One story might help illustrate some of the ways we would help out with Pop's random business ideas. I was about eight years old, and walking home from school one day. I stopped by the office, and Pop had one of those motorized carts that they have at the mall for senior citizens or people with disabilities. He was thinking about buying one as an investment, so he asked if I wanted to drive it home to "test it out." Reluctantly, I accepted, but I felt really awkward about the whole thing. As I drove this cart down Chester Avenue, I hit a bumpy patch around tree roots on the sidewalk, and I nearly tipped the thing over because you need to let go to stop it. But something in my mind was thinking I should pull it harder, and it sped up. Then I remember thinking, "Oh my gosh, people driving by are probably thinking this person with a disability needs help." And then all the traffic quickly stopped across Chester Avenue! I was horrified. Pop never did buy it!

Jackie: Our parents absolutely shared stories with us about clients and challenges, and we saw the aides firsthand come in to take care of Grandmom. Ultimately, this helped shape the kind of adult I would become and the path I would choose. It eventually became my turn to share stories about my patients at the dinner table.

Kelli: It was really neat to be so aware of and involved with your parents' work. I remember seeing their passion for nursing, for home care, and for just simply helping people who need help—both at the company and in the community—and that certainly left an indelible mark on me. I also remember the very special relationships they, and we, had with people at the company. It was a very close-knit group.

Christin: It was stressful for Mark and Mommy, I'm sure, juggling five kids and two full-time, demanding jobs, but I don't remember feeling stressed. They did such a good job of handling it all and keeping the family together and fun!

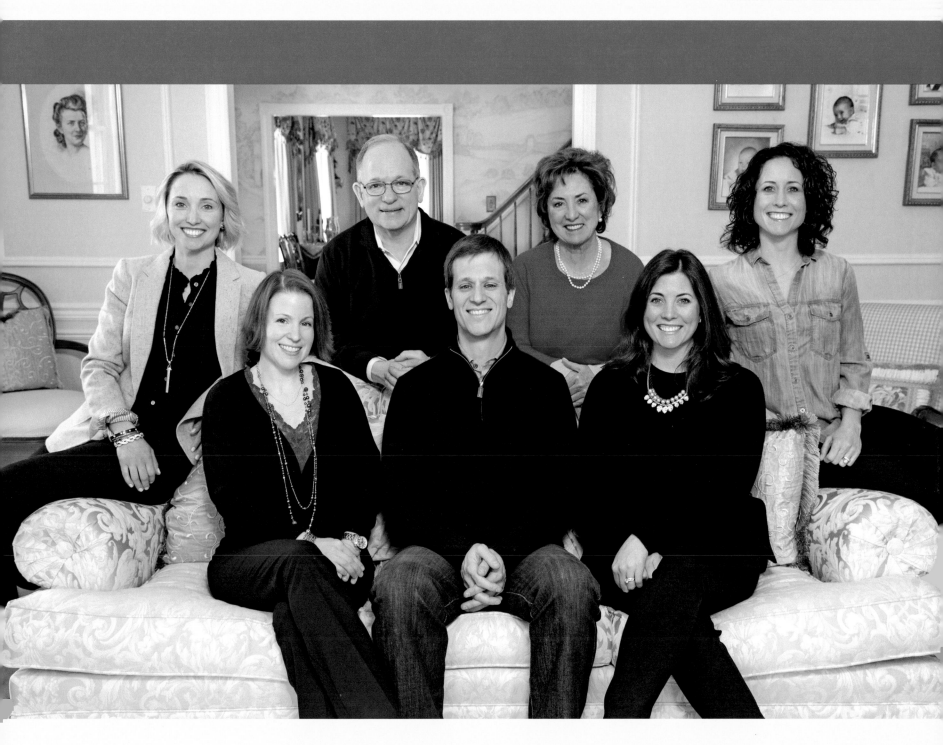

OUR VALUES

P2
1/8/2005
Al F.

#1 Value: *Compassion*

Key Result: We develop and maintain supportive and caring long-term relationships that make a substantial difference in the lives of the people we touch.

Key Actions: Work exceptional

1. Living with a spirit of hope, faith, and love.
2. Demonstrating care for our clients, for each other, and our community.
3. Communicating with each other clearly, honestly, and thoughtfully. ③ Listen closely + show empathy.
4. Treating people the way they want to be treated.
5. Finding and affirming the good in each other and what we do.

#2 Value: *Reliability*

Key Result: Our clients rely on us and live their lives to the fi— well-being, dignity, and trust.

Key Actions:
1. Delivering the expected services better than any other pro—
2. Keeping our commitments.
3. Always showing up as promised.
4. Be determined — get the job done.
5. Communicate clearly ...

#3 Value: *Excellence*

Key Result: We consistently get the job done for our clients at ethical, performance, and professional standards.

Key Actions: Commitment,
1. Exhibiting honesty and loyalty with our clients, each oth—
2. Consistently demonstrating a high level of skill, compete— in our work.
3. Making prudent and effective use of our time, money and
4. Working hard. + efficiently. our work.
5. Continuously improving at what we do.

Ann Baiada — So here we go to our first office for the "Bayada Way" tour. For this trip, it is me, Mark + Andrew Gentile. Andrew has been a terrific help for all of this + I wonder what we would do without him!

I feel excited that this is finally happening! I feel nervous about the size of the vehicle. Mark looks a bit nervous as well — especially at the toll booth on the Betsy Ross Bridge! I guess it will take some time to get used to it. It is huge!

This means the world to Mark and I feel good of him. He is a good man and a good boss. He cares so much about his employees and really wants to make a difference in this world.

We're off!

Andrew Gentile — The Bayada Way Tour has begun! I can't believe that we are driving in a 38ft RV on our way to

Sat, Jan 8th
2005
AmF

Draft: 1/4/05
Al Freedman

THE BAYADA WAY

OUR MISSION

Bayada Nurses have a special purpose—to help people have a safe home life with comfort, independence, and dignity, (despite illness or disability).

More families prefer to cope with illness or disability in their own homes. They like the privacy, the freedom, the familiar surroundings. Family and friends are closer.

Families often need help and support in caring for someone at home. They need *compassionate*, *reliable*, and *excellent* health care. These are the Bayada Nurses values—*compassion*, *reliability*, and *excellence*.

Bayada Nurses help with skilled nursing, personal care, therapy, meals, laundry, homemaking, and companionship. They help 24 hours a day, seven days a week—on any schedule.

Bayada Nurses' goals are to give the finest home care service available to families in need, to be recognized and respected for the important work they do, and to help more people who need care in their homes.

OUR VISION

To create a lasting legacy as the world's most dedicated and trusted home health care

---

September 2
Wayne, PA

Bonnie Lang

Judy Steinel

Etta DiMarco — a way to go.

Maryellen

Maria Bellochis

LEFT: Finalizing the words of *The BAYADA Way* took nine months and 23 drafts.

ABOVE: Number one of a series of journals from *The BAYADA Way* bus tour. It was Ann Baiada's idea to have employees at each stop record their thoughts in writing. Ann's own entry was the first.

"People can say that no one is irreplaceable, but Mark is irreplaceable. There's not another Mark and there won't be. He's so humble and so kind and so good. He's an inspiration."
ANN BAIADA

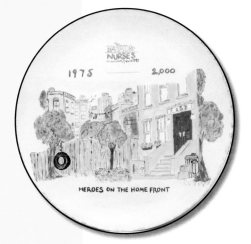

ABOVE: Pat Lefton, a Philadelphian who directed one of the first Florida offices, handcrafted this ceramic plate as a gift to the Baiadas.

The year 2000 marked a new millennium and the twenty-fifth year of BAYADA Nurses. For several years prior, office employees from across the country had congregated annually for a day of continuing education sessions followed by a dinner. There was plenty of warmth and camaraderie, but for the silver anniversary, Mark thought bigger. Harkening back to the "work hard, play hard" ethic of earlier years, he wanted the special get-together to emphasize recognition, celebration, gratitude, and sheer fun.

Cris Toscano, a Division Director based in Parsippany, New Jersey, vividly remembers both kinds of events. Very soon after she joined the company in 1994, Cris attended the smaller yearly session. "My most memorable moment

2001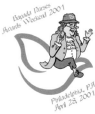

2002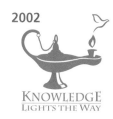

2005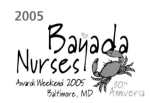

2008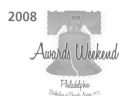

2009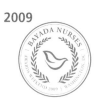

2010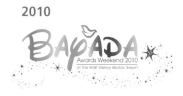

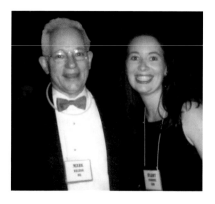

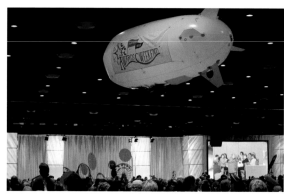

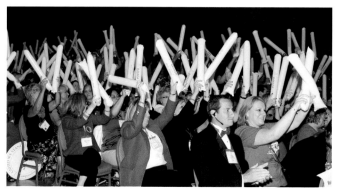

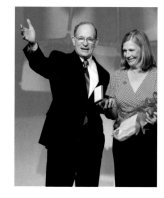

TOP ROW: Mark, after dyeing his hair green to celebrate a billings record, with Hilary Osborne in 2004.

A remote-controlled blimp flew over attendees in 2013.

BOTTOM ROW: Spirited employees cheering at the 2012 Awards Weekend with inflatable clappers.

BAYADA celebrates Years of Service. Here, Carol Elliott is awarded for 25 years.

of my whole time at BAYADA comes from that first event," she says. "At the end everyone stood in a circle and started singing 'That's What Friends Are For.' At first I thought, 'What? I'm not sure if I'm going to like working here. I'm not sure.' I knew people were very connected to each other. Then I realized they felt this deep connection and I thought, oh my gosh. That was the moment when I said, 'Okay, this is where I want to be.' These are people you want to work with forever, but not just that—they're people who become

your friends." (That song about friendship, by the way, is a very special one in the company's history. Thousands of other employees have sung it often and felt those feelings deeply every time.)

Memorable too, as Cris says, were the years when "literally every person at the yearly events could join hands in a big circle, because there weren't that many of us." The Awards Weekend of 2000 symbolized the sheer growth of the company. BAYADA had reached a size and level of success that warranted a major event at Disney World—the ideal place for fun, and a fitting backdrop for a bounty of blessings well worth celebrating. The company had grown from an idea into a thriving organization that had made a difference to hundreds of thousands of clients and their families. In the previous decade alone, it had more than doubled its offices to a total of 45 U.S. locations.

Strictly as an event, the weekend at Disney World raised the bar for the future. Awards Weekends have evolved into eagerly anticipated extravaganzas that emphasize camaraderie and recognition. Many office employees cite them as among their most memorable BAYADA memories.

The time had passed when every person at a yearly event could physically stand in a single circle and join hands. Yet BAYADA's philosophy—traditionally understood and shared mostly by word-of-mouth—had not changed. To keep it alive, however, it had to be articulated and better communicated to thousands of new field and office employees. That process became a priority. It would not be straightforward or easy, but Mark knew instinctively that it could not be hurried.

2011

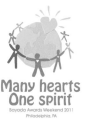

Many hearts
One spirit
Bayada Awards Weekend 2011
Philadelphia, PA

2013

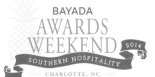

BAYADA
2013
HERSHEY, PA
AWARDS WEEKEND

2014

BAYADA
AWARDS
WEEKEND 2014
SOUTHERN HOSPITALITY
CHARLOTTE, NC

2015

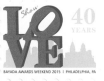

SHOW
LOVE 40 YEARS
BAYADA AWARDS WEEKEND 2015 | PHILADELPHIA, PA

LEFT: A selection of Awards Weekend logos from over the years.

Awards Weekend memories

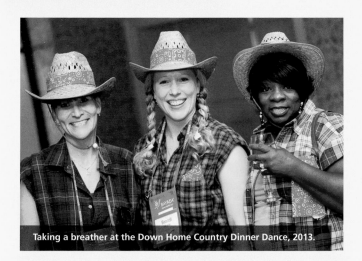

Taking a breather at the Down Home Country Dinner Dance, 2013.

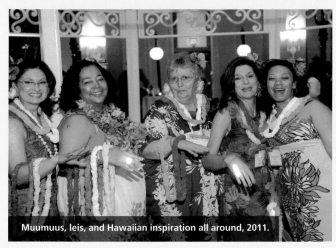

Muumuus, leis, and Hawaiian inspiration all around, 2011.

A major highlight of each year, Awards Weekend celebrates the hard work of everyone at BAYADA. It encourages connections and common purpose, which are so important to nurture as the company grows.

"I remember my first Awards Weekend, the company's silver anniversary at Disney World. My whole family came. The fact that Mark would honor all the office employees made the event feel small and family-oriented, even though it was large," says Karen Rizzo, RN, MS and Division Director, Home Care Division in Tucson, Arizona.

The spirit reenergizes employees, too. "When you head home, you're reconnected and reengaged," says Melinda Phillips, Division Director of the Home Health Specialty Practice in Salisbury, North Carolina. "If you were losing some of your steam, it's a good way to get your steam back."

A typically joyful moment emblazoned in many memories is the Hams and Fans dinner dance of 2004, which encouraged guests to don costumes, crazy hats, or headpieces. (Mark coined the phrase: "Hams are those who love the spotlight and Fans are those who love to watch them.") At this one, Mark spray-dyed his hair kelly green in honor of Kermit the Frog, his alter ego, and wore a bowtie to match. As he and everyone else enjoyed his verdant look, Mark realized it is easy being green.

The deepest feelings abound during Hero Awards presentations. "A lot of times during the awards, I get so emotional I have to leave the room," says Joanne Wilson, currently a Director working in the Home Care Technology office. "Awards Weekend is a very emotional gathering—we do a lot of smiling, laughing, and crying."

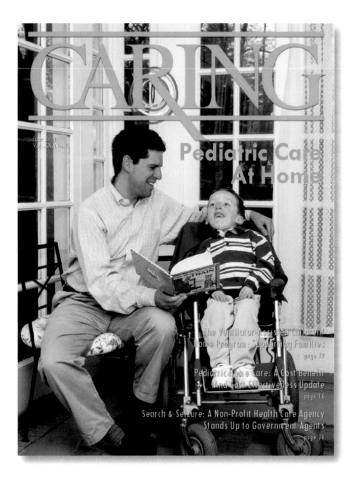

Connecting with Al Freedman

Serendipity or fate intervened when Mark happened to read a poignant essay by psychologist and father Albert (Al) Freedman, PhD, called "Welcome to Our Home," in the June 2001 issue of *CARING* magazine. Al wrote the piece as a thank-you letter to the professionals who cared for his son, Jack. At six months old, Jack had been diagnosed with spinal muscular atrophy, a degenerative and incurable condition. Doctors had told the Freedmans that Jack would live at most for a year, yet the boy had already surpassed that prediction. In the article, Al explained in detail what life is like for a family with a medically fragile child and spoke from the heart about the ups and downs of having health care professionals constantly in his home. The piece moved Mark and Ann deeply.

BAYADA reached out to Al by phone and invited him to speak at the annual Awards Weekend in Princeton, New Jersey, in June 2002. Surprised, he agreed. That weekend Al spoke about Jack and his experience from a parent's perspective, making a similarly strong impression on the audience. Mark approached Al privately and said he thought that Al could help him with something important at BAYADA. But he didn't specify what.

Al picks up the story: "I said, 'Sure, your nurses are helping with Jack, so of course I'd be happy to help you.' But I didn't quite know what he was thinking about." A few months later, Mark and Al met again. "I thought Mark wanted me to do more workshops for BAYADA employees, so I wrote out a plan with a list of potential workshop topics. I remember coming in to his office with

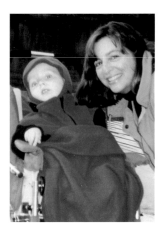

ABOVE: Baby Jack Freedman and his first BAYADA nurse, Wendy. At BAYADA's fortieth anniversary, Jack has defied the odds and is now 20 years old. He remains medically fragile, but with the support of his parents and BAYADA Nurses, Jack goes to school, uses a computer, and continues to charm everyone who meets him.

LEFT: The article and photos featured in the June 2001 issue of *CARING* magazine led to the life-changing relationship between the Freedmans and BAYADA.

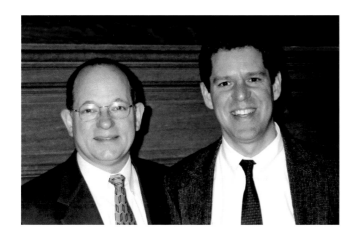

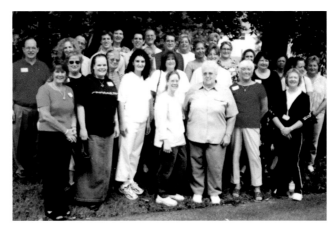

my neatly typed, two-page plan, trying to show him that I was conscientious. Mark took a very quick look at it, and he just turned it upside down and put it on the table. I thought to myself, 'Well, I guess that's not what he wants me to help with.'"

Mark wanted Al's help with a bigger idea. "He told me, 'Al, I've been thinking about 100 years from now. I've been thinking about what will happen when I'm gone. I want to make sure that in 100 years, someone like you, who has a child like Jack, will be able to get the same kind of help you're getting now. I need to write down who we are and what we stand for and what we believe in at BAYADA, so people will know what to do when I'm gone.'"

In his visionary way, Mark also talked about the legacies of Mother Teresa, Martin Luther King, Jr., and Florence Nightingale. Like others who have been surprised by Mark's sudden leaps of thought, Al admits, "I remember thinking

to myself, 'This guy's a little crazy.' Then I reminded myself that I'm a psychologist. I'm trained for this kind of stuff. So I did a lot of listening. As I listened to Mark, I realized how deeply he cared about clients like my son and that he meant every word he said. I sensed very quickly that Mark wasn't kidding when he said he was thinking 100 years into the future."

Mark circled back to his point: "I want to write down what we believe in, like the founding fathers did with the Declaration of Independence. I think you can help me do this. Would you be willing to write this for me?"

Just before saying yes, Al confessed bluntly: "I've never done anything like this before." Mark's response was, "That's okay—neither have I." It was Al's first encounter with a classic BAYADA figure-it-out sea wall situation. "That neither of us has ever done anything like this before is a running joke with us now," laughs Al.

"*I had the honor of being the emcee at our Awards Weekend in Atlantic City, a very special one because it's where we announced* The BAYADA Way *project. It was the first time everyone got to meet Al Freedman and hear his story. Al and his son Jack are such a profound part of the BAYADA family.*"

MARIE BLESSINGTON, RN, who started in 1985 and is Director of Clinical Leadership Development at the Clinical Standards and Quality office

TOP LEFT: Mark and Al Freedman in 2003.

TOP RIGHT: Participants at *The BAYADA Way* retreat, held at Pendle Hill in Wallingford, Pennsylvania, in 2004. This was the first of three retreats in which the actual writing of the document began.

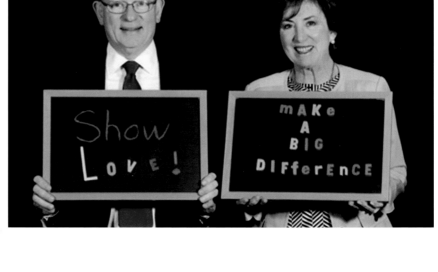

RIGHT: Core values, displayed by Mark and Ann for a pediatric video.

BELOW RIGHT: More than 5,500 employees and clients answered values-related surveys.

BELOW: An exercise done at *The BAYADA Way* retreats in 2004 that helped define the company's values.

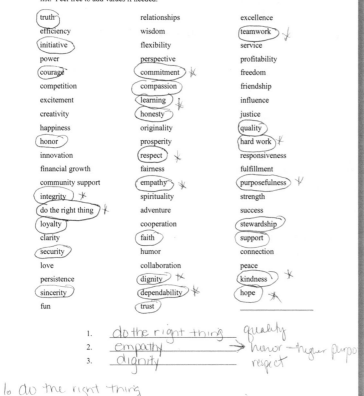

OUR VALUES

What should Bayada Nurses stand for? What should be the values by which we operate? Look over the list of values below. Circle any values that "jump out" because of their importance to you. Then write your *top three* values in order of importance, below the list. Feel free to add values if needed.

truth · efficiency · initiative · power · courage · competition · excitement · creativity · happiness · honor · innovation · financial growth · community support · integrity · do the right thing · loyalty · clarity · security · love · persistence · sincerity · fun

relationships · wisdom · flexibility · perspective · commitment · compassion · learning · honesty · originality · prosperity · respect · fairness · empathy · spirituality · adventure · cooperation · faith · humor · collaboration · dignity · dependability · trust

excellence · teamwork · service · profitability · freedom · friendship · influence · justice · quality · hard work · responsiveness · fulfillment · purposefulness · strength · success · stewardship · support · connection · peace · kindness · hope

1. do the right thing   quality
2. empathy → honor — higher purpo
3. dignity   respect

1. do the right thing
2. honor — higher purpose — code of behavior character

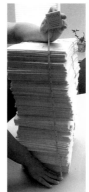

"Showing love and having faith"

The rest, one might say, is BAYADA history. In many companies, mission statements and core-values exercises fall flat because they don't connect with the work of front-line employees. There was no danger of that at BAYADA, because Al and Mark wanted the philosophy to be defined by the people "closest to the action"—the ones who do the actual work and live the company's values every day.

Al came aboard as a consultant. From 2002 to 2004, he met regularly with Mark and Baiada family members, nurses, aides, office employees, Directors, and Division Directors. A typical focus group would involve a mix of up to 15 people who met for 90 minutes. Like any good psychologist, Al probed for their true feelings, in this case about their work: What led you to choose the work you do? What does it look like when things are going well in a client's home? How does it feel to you when you're making a difference in someone's life? What should BAYADA stand for and believe in? What are the values that BAYADA holds as sacred? Al also spoke with clients and their families about their experiences.

"I heard a lot, especially from our nurses and aides, about showing love and having the faith that you're going to make a difference in someone's life," says Al. The ability to "show love" with clients resonated strongly with Mark, who had learned the phrase at his first orientation session as a volunteer in 1980 at Samaritan Hospice in southern New Jersey.

After gathering a wealth of responses, Al and Mark led three 24-hour retreats with 75 participants from all parts of the organization. The goal was to begin creating a written statement. "We deliberated on the concepts that should be part of *The BAYADA Way*," says Al. "I led the group through different exercises to help clarify what the document should include." These groups narrowed down 40 values to eight, enabling the company to develop a survey that was sent to every client and employee—about 19,000 people. More than 5,500 replied, an extremely high response rate.

With the philosophy well refined, the next step was to write it. Al drafted the document at the foot of Jack's bed, while his 9-year-old son was sleeping. "Back then, I was Jack's night nurse three nights a week," says Al. "I'd get Jack out of his wheelchair, bathe and dress him, get him into bed, plug in his feeding pump, put on his breathing mask, and get all the machines and monitors turned on. Then I would work for a couple of hours on my laptop before I got some sleep in the other bed in Jack's room. Jack's presence helped me to stay focused and aware of the importance of each and every word I was writing."

Paying it forward

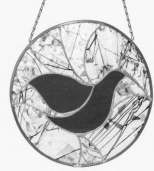

For many years, BAYADA employees generously showed their appreciation to Mark and Ann by sending gifts at Christmas and other times of the year. Although the Baiadas were deeply grateful, they felt the money could be better spent helping others.

After Mark discussed his concerns with Joanne Wilson, former Accounting Supervisor and currently a Director working in Home Care Technology, they came up with a plan. "We agreed to have a fund for employees in need," says Joanne. "We put out the word to employees that instead of a gift, they could put money into the BAYADA Emergency Fund."

Since 2001, the Emergency Fund has helped employees who have experienced difficulties caused by the unexpected job loss of a spouse, fires, natural disasters, medical, and other emergencies. For legal reasons, the donated funds can't pay for medical bills or medications, but they assist greatly with utility bills, rent, and other financial needs. Following the Fund's success, the company created The BAYADA Foundation as a nonprofit 501(c)3 charitable organization in 2011. It provides financial assistance to people in need and supports charitable causes or programs through two funds: the Employee and Client Emergency Fund and the Hospice Fund.

"This has been a great way to support our community and support *The BAYADA Way*," says Hilary Osborne, Senior Manager of Internal Communications.

"BAYADA employees instinctively want to help other BAYADA employees and clients in times of need. The funds enable us to do so and demonstrate BAYADA's desire to show love and demonstrate exceptional kindness."

Nine months and 23 drafts later, the company finalized the document and officially named it *The BAYADA Way*. It debuted at Awards Weekend 2005 in Baltimore, officially clarifying the mission, vision, beliefs, and values that were and continue to be the foundation of the company. It articulates three core values: compassion, excellence, and reliability. It also expresses that BAYADA employees "work with a spirit of universal faith, hope, and love."

Spreading the news

The fact remained that even the most thoughtfully crafted document isn't a living, breathing philosophy until it becomes part of daily work life. The question became how to share and sustain *The BAYADA Way* across the organization. Each office received written copies and a video. Yet Mark felt it needed to be further personalized.

For many years, almost everyone had reported directly to Mark. For years after that, he made it his business to meet and remember the name of virtually every employee. Understandably, those days were over, and many newer employees knew him and Ann only through hearing stories about them, seeing them on video, or meeting them briefly at an orientation or training session. Unveiling *The BAYADA Way* in person, the Baiadas realized, would provide an ideal way to connect meaningfully and show love, office by office. Sitting around a table with employees, laughing and sharing a meal, talking about compassion, excellence, and reliability—this all felt just right.

If properly used, the philosophy would have another benefit: it would help BAYADA maintain its small-company

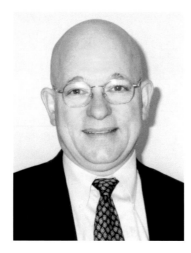

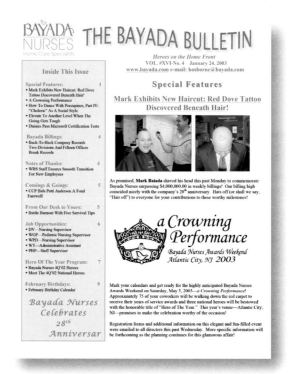

feeling. "Sometimes you're working in a business and you feel you're all on your own," Mark says. "This way we could feel closer to others—more support, more that we were all part of the same, big team."

Make no mistake: Mark still did this in ways big and small. In 2003, for example, he made a New Year's resolution to shave his head when BAYADA surpassed $4 million in weekly billings. The company reached that milestone during a January week so cold that the Delaware River had almost frozen, but Mark kept his wacky promise. What's more, after the barber shaved his head, something peculiar emerged on Mark's scalp: a red BAYADA dove tattoo.

"Mark had someone draw the dove there and take a photo of it to share with the whole company," says wife Ann, who made him wear a hat until his hair grew back. "All these crazy ideas are Mark's!"

LEFT: Mark's wacky way of celebrating $4 million in weekly billings came just in time for Awards Weekend 2003.

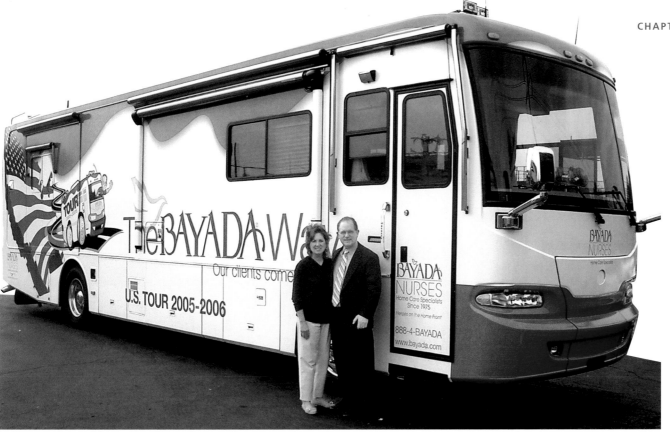

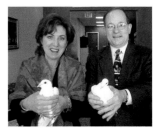

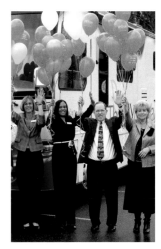

Birth of the bus

In a nod to his fondness for *The Muppet Movie*, where like-minded characters travel on a bus to bigger things, Mark decided on a bus tour, too. He first considered using a school bus like the one Kermit drove. "Then Mark came up with what he thought was an even better idea," reminisces Andrew Gentile, who was Mark's tour apprentice at the time and is now Home Health Operating Policy Director. "He wanted an old Volkswagen van. You know, peace, love, and all that!"

The tour committee gently reminded Mark that Ann would often be traveling with him, and that she might notice the lack of modern-day comforts in an old VW van. Ann is a trouper, but driving without air-conditioning through Florida or Arizona—or even Philadelphia on a humid day—can test the patience of even the most devoted couple. Like any sensible husband, Mark reconsidered.

The committee settled on a comfortable tour bus, wrapped "rock band" style with the BAYADA logo, a cartoon image of Mark driving the bus, and a photo of Nurse Lisa from the company's iconic TV commercial on the back.

Sherri Pillet, a 35-year BAYADA veteran who is Division Director of the Employee Relations and was on the Bus Tour committee, explains: "We felt like if we wrapped the RV, we'd be able to share that spirit everywhere we went." That's exactly what happened. Mark and Ann, sometimes with Al or other guests, would ultimately visit 124 offices in 15 states to help everyone "get on the bus" of *The BAYADA Way*.

LEFT: The bus traveled across the country to 124 offices.

TOP: Ann and Mark preparing for a symbolic dove release on one of their stops along the tour.

ABOVE: A warm welcome in Asheville, North Carolina. Exuberant employees greeted the tour at every stop.

What it means to be on the BAYADA bus

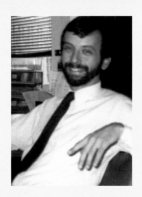

David Roarty wrote and shared the following document in November 2003. At that time, he was Director of the Personal Care Assistant Office in Philadelphia. A beloved employee since 1979, David was "a stalwart of our early motley crew of *Muppet Movie*-like characters pursuing our worthy common goal to make it to our Hollywood," says Mark. David passed away in 2011 and is fondly remembered for his feisty "must do" spirit and unrelenting dedication to excellence.

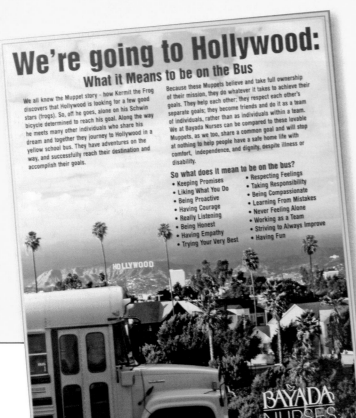

ABOVE LEFT AND RIGHT: David in the 1980s; David and Mark on stage at Awards Weekend in 2010.

LEFT: David's words adapted for a poster.

OPPOSITE TOP LEFT: Artwork created during the Bus Tour by three support offices: Managed Care (MCO), Insurance Confirmation (ICO), and Contract Management (CMO).

OPPOSITE TOP RIGHT: The Bus Tour inspired lots of employee creativity.

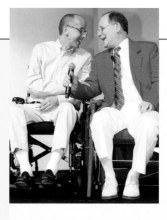

What it means to be on the BAYADA bus
Shared by David Roarty, Director, PCA

We all know the Muppet story: How Kermit the Frog, alone in a swamp, discovers that Hollywood is looking for a few good frogs. He decides he wants to be a star with a little encouragement from Dom DeLuise. So off he goes, alone on his Schwinn bicycle, determined to reach his goal. Along the way, he meets many other similar-minded individuals who share his dream and together they journey to Hollywood in a yellow school bus. They have adventures on the way, and successfully reach their destination and accomplish their goals.

Because these Muppets believe and take full ownership of their mission, they do whatever it takes to achieve their goals. They help each other; they respect each other's separate goals; they become friends and do it as a team of individuals, rather than individuals within a team.

We at BAYADA Nurses can be compared to these lovable Muppets, as we too, share a common goal and will stop at nothing to help people have a safe home life with comfort, independence, and dignity, despite illness or disability.

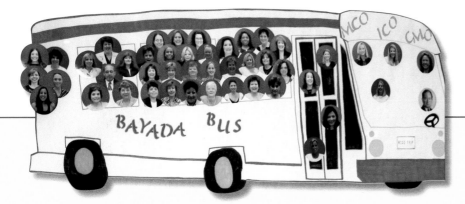

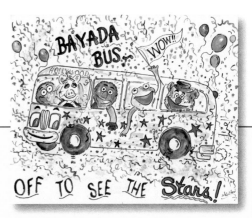

So what does it really mean to be "on the bus"?

To me, it means:

- **Keeping promises.** Always keeping your promises and never promising anything that you cannot honestly deliver. Staying late and/or taking an employee's or consumer's phone number home to call them—only because you promised you would get back to them that day.

- **Truly liking what you do,** so that it shows in every call and/or contact with all employees and consumers whether it is 9:00 AM or 4:57 PM.

- **Being proactive,** even though it may cause extra work for you.

- **Having courage** and being brave enough when asking an employee whose schedule is already maxed out to do that extra shift (which you know she will probably take) when that employee is one of your very few options to cover the shift and saying at the end: "Please say no if you really don't want to" knowing full well that she may take you up on it and decline.

- Taking the time to **really listen** to both your employees and consumers.

- To absolutely never think of an employee as simply a warm body or someone with "availability" and to never think of consumers as simply an address. **Remember we are dealing with people.**

- To realize that your employees do **give their all** when providing service and to also give your all (complete and accurate directions; honestly advise them of what they may be walking into, etc.).

- **Never lying** under any circumstances and never embellishing anything to make life easier for you. Never shift blame where it doesn't belong.

- Making a decent **attempt to understand** where that "challenged" consumer/caregiver may be coming from whether you agree or not. By listening, you will validate his/her feelings.

- **Being compassionate.** To always remember that behind every single "challenge" is a little scared person needing help. To strive to make your best effort in accepting people as they are and not as you think they should be.

- **Respecting feelings.** Realize that the homebound consumer's world, unlike yours, is limited and challenging. What may not seem very important to us may be extremely important to them.

- **Working as a team.** Be aware of your fellow workers' jobs and responsibilities and strive to help—even when you are busy yourself.

- **Taking responsibility** for your work, and remembering to ask for help when needed and to return that favor when asked by others.

- **Having fun** doing this important and stressful and energy-zapping work. Create a serious, yet warm and human atmosphere within the office.

- **Learning from your mistakes**, and getting right back on the bus—not beating yourself up.

- **Making a huge fuss over your employees** from your heart.

- Leaving your own personal problems at the door—to actually say to yourself **"SHOW TIME"** before walking into your office or whatever "mantra" works for you. Decide to have a **positive attitude** no matter what.

- **Never feeling alone,** because you are not— you are **"on the bus."**

Being on the bus is a state of mind— enjoy the ride! 🌿

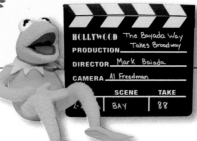

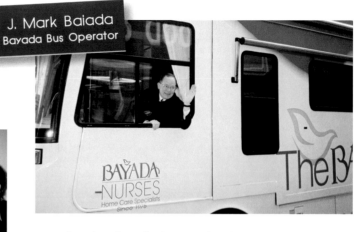

On the road in earnest

An Oregon vendor had the best price on the 38-foot motor home that matched the specs for the BAYADA bus. David Baiada and his wife Mindy, who love to travel, picked it up there and drove it back East. The official road trip started in September 2005. It wasn't one continuous journey, because Mark and Ann couldn't be away from the office for unbroken stretches. It happened in phases, with Bonnie Carr Long, retired Manager of Special Projects, and Andrew Gentile expertly orchestrating the logistics.

A couple of the initial trips involved navigating downtown Philadelphia with Andrew onboard. Only a commercial truck driver would be comfortable squeezing a 38-foot motor home through some of the city's narrow old streets, yet Mark insisted on doing it himself. As they turned a corner one day, Andrew heard a noise. "Uh oh, Mark, we just clipped that parked car." Andrew immediately ran to the car and left an apologetic note with contact information. All expenses for damage repair were paid.

The tour took place in segments, with *The BAYADA Way* consultant Al Freedman, PhD, often joining in. At each stop, BAYADA folks embraced the Baiadas with a bounty of food, gifts, and locally inspired welcome ceremonies. Mark gained 15 pounds along the way, but every ounce was worthwhile. "The offices started trying to one-up each other," says Andrew. Among the 124 office greetings for the BAYADA bus tour:

- Denver office employees performed a Native American ceremony complete with incense, smoke, headdresses, and drumbeats.

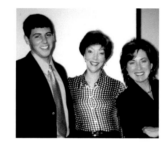

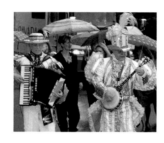

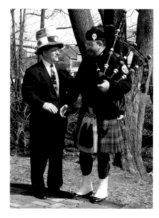

TOP TO BOTTOM: Tour orchestrators Andrew Gentile and Bonnie Long with Ann.

Musical greetings in Pennsylvania from the Mummers in Willow Grove and a bagpiper in Newtown.

- In the City of Brotherly Love, the Philadelphia Eagles' mascot Swoop hugged them; in nearby Willow Grove, a lively Mummers string band played.

- At the Salisbury, North Carolina office, an employee costumed as a classic Southern belle (think Scarlett O'Hara in *Gone with the Wind*) waited on the sidewalk in her flowing violet gown and parasol to greet them.

- The Accounting office employees put down their Excel spreadsheets and formed a cheerleading squad.

- Bagpipers rang out a Scottish welcome in Newtown, Pennsylvania.

- In Winston-Salem, North Carolina, the employees had real doves—a key element of the BAYADA logo—on hand for the Baiadas to release into the sky.

- Anna Anderson of the Morristown, New Jersey, office wrote a BAYADA poem to the theme of *'Twas the Night Before Christmas.*

- At the Communications office in New Jersey, a red carpet and conga line of employees greeted Mark and Ann, where they viewed an employee-made film of *The BAYADA Way* starring Senior Internal Communications Manager Hilary Osborne as Miss Piggy and Senior External Communications Manager Jim Armstrong as Mark's beloved Kermit.

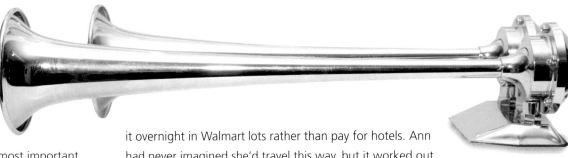

Sharing stories

Amidst all the fun and excitement, it was most important to Mark that the office employees truly "get" the message. At each office, the travelers spent at least half a day with employees. Mark spoke about *The BAYADA Way* and after viewing the poignant explanatory video, the groups spoke from the heart about their work and the company's vision. "Tears were flowing at every stop we made," says Andrew.

In a journal kept by Ann, she wrote about the first visit to the downtown Philadelphia office: "Everyone loved the bus! . . . We listened to Mark's presentation and watched the video—not a dry eye was in the room. Mark did a great job explaining his beliefs and how important this all is to him." Many more tears of gratitude would be shed; poems and thank-you notes would be written.

Often employees shared their own experiences with family members or friends who led them to work in home health care. They told stories of parents, children, siblings, grandparents, and uncles and aunts who had faced or were facing health challenges and needed help. Some employees revealed that they chose to work at BAYADA to honor the memories of family members or friends who had passed away.

"Just as it was not a coincidence that I was led to BAYADA, it was not a coincidence for a number of our office employees to join BAYADA," says Al. "And our tour stops provided the opportunity for everyone involved to 'connect to our purpose' by sharing those stories."

The motor home was comfortable enough to sleep in, which meant BAYADA Bus drivers could economically park it overnight in Walmart lots rather than pay for hotels. Ann had never imagined she'd travel this way, but it worked out fine. Karen Rizzo, MS, RN, and Division Director in Tucson, Arizona, remembers that her little daughter was fascinated by the whole idea. "So we went over to the Walmart lot before school and took a picture of her by the bus," says Karen. "It was really cool."

Employees also noticed the humility of the Baiadas. Here were company leaders who camped overnight with other RV owners. Mark drove the bus himself, gleefully honking the big horn whenever the opportunity arose. Westerners especially appreciated that the president would journey thousands of miles west, across lonely stretches of highway, rather than just hopping on a plane.

The tour culminated at the spring 2006 Awards Weekend in New York City. Having lived in Manhattan, David Baiada volunteered to pilot the bus along crowded 42nd Street to the Marriott Marquis Hotel. The journey had succeeded. Even jaded Manhattanites stopped to look as the bus made its climactic journey to the 2006 Awards Weekend.

ABOVE: Sounding the double horn was one of Mark's favorite parts of driving the bus. The horn is on display at Headquarters.

BOTTOM LEFT: Smiles abounded at the Wilmington (Delaware) office.

BOTTOM RIGHT: David Baiada piloted the bus to its last official stop, the 2006 Awards Weekend in New York City.

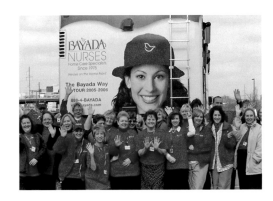

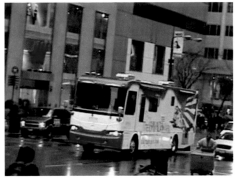

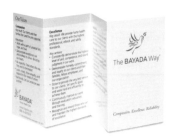

ABOVE: Small wallet card with a big impact.

BELOW: Ongoing advocacy efforts include events such as the annual BAYADA Day at the state capitol building in Harrisburg, Pennsylvania.

Embedded philosophy radiates outward

Everyone was on board with *The BAYADA Way*. Those who couldn't embrace it tended to self-select out of the company—true for job seekers and new hires as well as a few longer-term employees.

"Everybody was talking about it. Everybody was part of it. Everybody felt the connection," says Bonnie Long. "Later, office employees implemented a fun training program so that the thousands of field employees could experience it, too." Printed onto a trim little four-fold laminated card, *The BAYADA Way* lives in employees' wallets and purses, on their desks, and in their hearts.

The philosophy has become culturally embedded. Interviewers ask candidates to talk about *The BAYADA Way*.

Office managers use *The BAYADA Way* exercises in weekly meetings. Every piece of communication cites a phrase or two, right down to signs in ladies' rooms that politely ask users to keep the sinks tidy. ("Be respectful," one such sign says, with paper towels helpfully stacked below.) Put into action daily, *The BAYADA Way* perpetuates itself.

"I'm always using it," says Melinda Phillips, whose favorite piece is "Treat others the way they wish to be treated." Such phrases, she notes, help to "remind people that it's not Melinda or whoever that's asking you to do this. It's the way our company operates. If you work here, this is expected."

Radiating outward, *The BAYADA Way* infuses every area the company touches, not the least of which is government policy and legislation. Because BAYADA works to provide the highest quality of care given by compassionate individuals, it advocates for policies in line with that philosophy. In fact, since 2009, the company's Government Affairs Office (GAO) has worked for the rights of home care clients and their families, in addition to home care employees on the local, state, and federal levels. GAO officials and volunteer employees called "ambassadors" have made a difference in scores of legislative issues. Efforts include a special website that makes it simple for employees to follow the latest news and get in touch with state and federal legislators to make a difference.

"The team I work with is considered one of the most innovative groups of government affairs advocates in the entire home health care industry," proudly states David Totaro, BAYADA's Chief Marketing and Government Affairs officer. "We have five political action committees, which is well more than average."

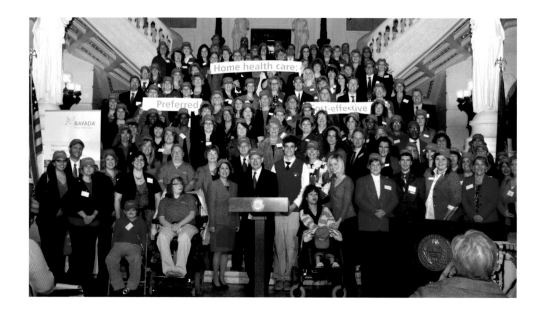

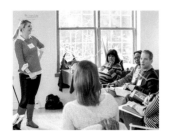

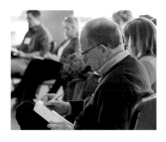

TOP: Employees regularly share ideas on putting *The BAYADA Way* into action.

ABOVE: Mark taking notes at one of *The BAYADA Way* retreats held in 2014.

"A much better version of myself"

"Working at BAYADA" is an oxymoron to most of the company's employees. It doesn't feel like work when you're making a difference doing something you love, with people you care about and values that you never have to compromise. Many say *The BAYADA Way* has helped make them better people all around.

"Working here has made me softer," says Sharon Vogel, Director of Hospice Services. "I used to be a much tougher person and less patient. I expected a lot out of others. I still do, but when I hit a rough patch, I think about *The BAYADA Way*: Would my responding this way really be consistent with it? Then, I follow it."

Tom Sibson, Central Support Services Practice Leader and Chief Financial and Administrative Officer, worked in a very cut-throat industry before joining BAYADA. "Working here has allowed me to be myself, which took a while for me to learn. I am more like I am at home as a father and a husband: more compassionate, more understanding, more sensitive, more tuned into what people need," says Tom. "My wife tells me all the time it's the best thing that ever happened to me and maybe her, too."

Company veteran Tom Mylet puts it succinctly: "The opportunities that BAYADA and Mark have afforded me have made me a much better version of myself."

What's more, the company's high standards consistently inspire employees to do better. "I feel like BAYADA has brought out the best in me and continued to reinforce the best in me. I think that comes from our strong culture of doing the right thing, always. That's the expectation

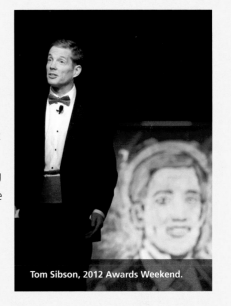

Tom Sibson, 2012 Awards Weekend.

and the norm," says Linda Siessel, Chief Operating Officer, Home Care Services, in Morristown, New Jersey. "I feel really, really grateful. I never have to feel ashamed or compromised in my own ethics, because they are one and the same with the company's. It doesn't get better than this." 🌿

The BAYADA Way in action on a special Christmas Day

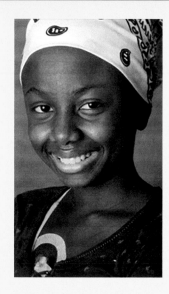

ABOVE: Siani spent her final Christmas with her family, in their own home, thanks to the dedication of BAYADA employees.

Fun and laughter boomed from the employees' holiday party at Voorhees Pediatrics in Voorhees, New Jersey. Then the phone rang. It was Children's Hospital of Philadelphia, familiarly known as CHOP. Mary Ellen Garofalo, Transitional Care Program Director, answered and quickly learned that a gravely ill 13-year-old girl, Siani, and her family had a wish to be home on Christmas Day and needed coverage.

Siani was so ill with leukemia that any attempt to move her could result in her death. She needed a nurse with the highest pediatric intensive care nursing skills.

December 25 was just days away. Having planned for coverage months in advance, Debra Magaraci, Director, learned of the situation and asked herself, "Who is available? All of our nurses were on shifts already."

But this was an extremely special circumstance. Siani's condition was terminal and this would likely be her last holiday at home. Without hesitation, Debra said to her office, "We're bringing this baby home. They can count on us."

Upon hearing the story, everyone at the party proceeded to make phone calls to nurses. One nurse offered to come off a complicated shift if someone else could fill in for her, so she could offer uninterrupted care to Siani.

Realizing that the family hadn't been home much—they'd been virtually living at CHOP—BAYADA employees dismantled the office Christmas tree, carried it to the family's home, and redecorated it there. Debra also called the local grocery store to have them cook and deliver a complete holiday dinner for the family.

Coming home and playing with the family dog one last time boosted Siani's spirits tremendously. "Her dad was walking around the house saying, 'I didn't know there were angels on earth. . . . I never knew there were angels,'" Debra says. "We cried all Christmas Day. It was a true Christmas miracle."

Educational advancements

In yet another vital area, employee education, BAYADA was poised to gain momentum. The "figure it out" approach had helped the company build many proverbial sea walls in the early years, but gone were the days of winging it. The company had constructed a solid foundation for learning in the 1980s and 1990s. By the 2000s it was in a strong financial position. What better way to invest in the future than to invest in learning?

Mark had been raised to believe that formal education was crucial to success, along with hands-on work experience. "My parents both understood the importance of education. My mom immigrated here and it didn't take long for her to figure out if you wanted to be successful, you needed an education," he says.

"Learning gives you the ability, which leads to competence. Then competence leads to confidence that ultimately leads to success."

Mark's love of education translated to increased professional development opportunities at every level. Piece by piece, the company added initiatives such as tuition reimbursement, the BAYADA Presidential Scholarship Program for employees, and webinars that took advantage of new learning technologies to transcend geography.

These efforts evolved into BAYADA University—the umbrella term for a host of initiatives that include two on-site learning centers (Burlington, New Jersey, and Charlotte, North Carolina), one-on-one instruction and preceptor models, self-directed learning, e-learning modules, and mentoring programs. Each new office employee attends

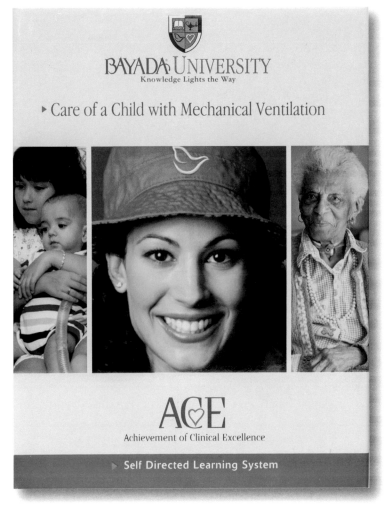

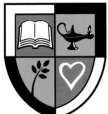

ABOVE: Clinical educational materials, early 2000s.

RIGHT: The BAYADA University seal encompasses formal learning, Florence Nightingale's iconic nursing lamp, a compassionate heart, and the BAYADA dove's olive branch.

"We established a fairly rigorous competency program for our employees who provide care to our clients who have tracheostomies or are on mechanical ventilation. At first, a few non-clinicians questioned why we needed to spend the time or the money to develop it. But within a few months after it was implemented, one of them said she realized that programs like this are what differentiate BAYADA as a company. Clinical excellence is the foundation."

BARBARA COLIN, MSN, RN, who started in 2001 and is Chief Nursing Officer, Moorestown, New Jersey

Welcome Training within the first few months of starting. Two popular programs specifically for nurses are Project White Cap, which offers BAYADA-specific initial training to all new clinical leaders, and Project White Shoes, an annual continuing education program for clinical leaders. These names derive from the white caps and shoes traditionally worn by nurses until the 1980s. BAYADA University includes a multitude of other on-site training and development courses for all office employees ranging from personal development to job-specific courses.

To promote a pipeline of future leaders, BAYADA established the Associate Leadership Development Program (ALDP). With support and training, the ALDP encourages recent college graduate employees who demonstrate competency necessary in management positions to move at least two levels within the company. Associates go through the six-month training ALDP program to become a Manager and, ultimately, a Director in two to five years. The program also attracts professionals in transition who resonate with *The BAYADA Way*. Usually these are people who have gained corporate experience elsewhere and want to make a difference in a more meaningful way.

"The ALDP gave me the tools and knowledge base to contribute to BAYADA's continued success. The training sessions offered were excellent and the exposure to the Management Committee was second to none. Since completing the ALDP, my career at BAYADA has been very rewarding. At BAYADA, you have a tremendous opportunity to make a positive impact on the lives of our clients and employees every day," shares Stephanie Kephart, who was

in the first graduating class in 2009. Today she is a service office Director in Kauai, Hawaii.

Because Mark feels so strongly about employee training, he likes to be present at much of it. As soon as web technology allowed, he began regularly speaking at webinars. He speaks in person at every Welcome Training session for new employees and ALDP training session for young leaders that take place at the New Jersey Learning Center in Burlington. For the sessions in Charlotte at the North Carolina Learning Center, Mark uses video conferencing technology to ensure new employees have the same experience. In fact, he organizes his schedule around the new employee training sessions, so he won't miss the opportunity to meet employees, talk about the history of BAYADA, and answer any questions they may have.

The alignment of BAYADA

The implementation of *The BAYADA Way* and the enhanced educational opportunities were an outgrowth of what BAYADA officially dubbed "the alignment." This broader idea was essentially a series of initiatives designed to align the company to the core values of *The BAYADA Way*.

Some background: Before writing *The BAYADA Way*, Mark and Al Freedman had read the book *Managing By Values*, written by Ken Blanchard and Michael O'Connor, PhD. Inspired by it and wanting further insight, they even arranged a meeting with O'Connor. "Dr. O'Connor says a company should be led by its values, not by people. So values are always on top," says Mark. The book's three main tenets helped to shape BAYADA's actions. First, the company had clarified values by developing *The BAYADA Way*. Second, it had communicated those values through the BAYADA bus tour. The third step was the alignment. These three steps are continuous—they don't just end with alignment. They're always being examined and implemented. Mark took to the stage at Awards Weekend 2006 to preview the initiatives that ultimately rolled out between 2008 and 2010.

"We made a strategic decision to work from a common, fundamental operating standard," says Central Support Services Practice Leader and Chief Financial and Administrative Officer Tom Sibson, who joined BAYADA in 2005. "*The BAYADA Way* gave us a common belief system, but not a common operating system. We recognized that if we're really going to grow, to scale up, we had to develop common methods and systems because replication is easier than starting every office organically."

One of the most significant initiatives included reorganizing the company into distinct and more formal specialty practices, known as *The BAYADA Way* of Organizing for Success. No longer would the company provide multiple specialties out of one office, organized by regions. Instead, offices were reorganized based on specialty, which helped streamline care.

David Baiada's experience in organizational structure, gained during an earlier job at a consulting firm, was instrumental. "We slowly started to carve out services and add a business unit within the company that had direct responsibility for providing some support services to these locations, in addition to what the organization provided overall," says David. "We were shifting BAYADA on its side a little bit by creating specialties instead of remaining organized by regions." At the company's fortieth anniversary, there are nine specialty practices at BAYADA Home Health Care. This enables BAYADA to provide a continuum of specialized services to clients across their lifespan. Organizing by specialty practice also enables the company to gain more expertise in specific types of services.

Like any corporate reorganization, the alignment raised fears. Would it entail layoffs? Why were outside consultants called in? Were other forces at work? Early in 2007, Mark assured Division Directors: "I will extinguish one rumor that is causing great distress. I will not sell BAYADA Nurses. Getting our house in order does not mean we want to sell

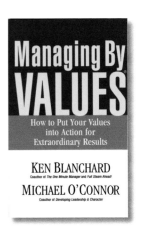

ABOVE: The inspirational book that guided Mark and Al while writing *The BAYADA Way*.

BELOW: An overview of alignment events from *The BAYADA Way* of Operating an Office, 2008.

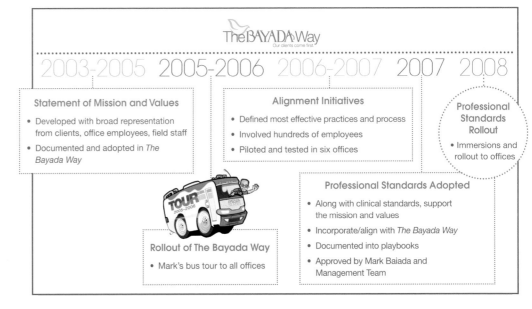

The BAYADA Way
Our clients come first

2003-2005 2005-2006 2006-2007 2007 2008

Statement of Mission and Values
- Developed with broad representation from clients, office employees, field staff
- Documented and adopted in *The Bayada Way*

Alignment Initiatives
- Defined most effective practices and process
- Involved hundreds of employees
- Piloted and tested in six offices

Professional Standards Rollout
- Immersions and rollout to offices

Rollout of The Bayada Way
- Mark's bus tour to all offices

Professional Standards Adopted
- Along with clinical standards, support the mission and values
- Incorporate/align with *The Bayada Way*
- Documented into playbooks
- Approved by Mark Baiada and Management Team

"There have been so many helpful trainings along the way, all these different years, but some of the most memorable were the Wave trainings. That was when we were aligning all the offices with the service lines, the policies, and such. Those were very helpful in terms of bringing everybody into alignment."

HOLLY WHITE, RN, VSN, who started in 1997 and is now Director, Staffing Office, Willow Grove, Pennsylvania

BAYADA Home Health Care specialty practices at a glance

• Home Health

BAYADA provides short-term nursing, rehabilitative, therapeutic, and assistive home health care services for adults and seniors. This care is provided as a limited number of up to one-hour visits primarily through the Medicare Home Health benefit.

• Adult Nursing

BAYADA provides nursing care services at home for adults of all ages dealing with chronic illness, injury, or disability. These services are provided primarily on an ongoing shift (two-hour or more) basis, and are available 24 hours a day, 7 days a week.

• Assistive Care

BAYADA provides non-medical assistance with activities of daily living, including self-care and household support services, for adults and seniors. These services are provided primarily on an ongoing shift (two-hour or more) basis, and are available 24 hours a day, 7 days a week.

• Assistive Care State Programs

BAYADA provides assistive care services (see above) paid for by state-sponsored contracts, Medicaid, Medicaid waiver, Managed Medicaid, or the Veterans benefits administration.

• Pediatrics

BAYADA provides nursing, therapeutic, and assistive home health care services for children under the age of 18, primarily on an ongoing shift (two-hour or more) basis. These services are available 24 hours a day, 7 days a week.

• Hospice

BAYADA provides comprehensive end-of-life clinical, social, emotional, and spiritual care that provides comfort and support to patients and their family members when a life-expectancy prognosis of six months or less has been determined. These services are available 24 hours a day, 7 days a week.

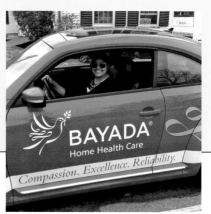

LEFT: Vermont Hospice team member Brigid Rice test-driving the beautiful BAYADA Bug owned by Division Director Maureen Hixon, who was visiting from Massachusetts.

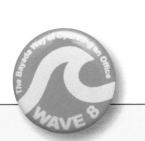

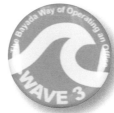
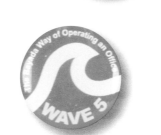
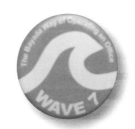

• Habilitation

BAYADA provides education, support, and assistance that enables clients with intellectual or developmental disabilities—including behavioral health—to acquire, maintain, and improve skills related to activities of daily living in order to function as meaningfully and independently as possible in the community. These services are available 24 hours a day, 7 days a week.

• Staffing

BAYADA provides qualified health care professionals to a variety of health care organizations, schools, medical practices, and other facilities for contract, per-diem, and temporary-to-permanent opportunities to assist with their staffing needs. These services are available 24 hours a day, 7 days a week.

• Central Support Services

The organizational name for the various internal offices that provide support services throughout the company in alignment with specific business objectives. These services offer a variety of high quality, cost effective, core services and consultative work. 🌿

ABOVE: *The BAYADA Way* of Operating an Office rolled out in eight Wave training sessions, commemorated with colorful pins.

it. On the contrary, it means we plan to live here permanently. . . . We've reorganized before, and we will again. The home health care market is evolving, and we have no choice but to accept. . . . Alignment is about putting the words of *The BAYADA Way* into action."

Also as part of the alignment initiative encouraging standardization, *The BAYADA Way* of Operating an Office rolled out in 2008. This regularly updated "playbook" uses the core philosophy to guide office policies and procedures, covering everything from the frequency of meetings to the exact shade of paint on the walls. "Just as we follow professional standards clinically, we needed to put them in place on the support side, to ensure that everything we're doing incorporates and aligns with *The BAYADA Way*," explains Hilary Osborne. Mark compares the result to an international presence such as Starbucks: their stores aren't identical, but they convey the same feeling and operate the same way from Seattle to Sarasota to Spain.

Additionally, in order for all the employees to be on board with alignment initiatives, BAYADA established "Wave" trainings. These consisted of eight uniform training modules to instruct employees on the new way of conducting BAYADA business. "The entire organization was in the same wave at the same time," says Tom. "The training progressed in a series from Wave 1 to Wave 8 over a few years."

Pediatric Specialty Practice Leader Karen Buttler, who joined BAYADA in 2003, puts the entire initiative and structure into elegant perspective. "As BAYADA continued to

grow—and we were growing by leaps and bounds—
we wanted to make sure that we were best in class in
every product we offered. Each Specialty Practice Leader
is responsible for supporting the vision of growth,
development, and innovation related to his or her product
line. Alignment is our effort to keep focused and provide
exceptional service, regardless of how large we get."
Karen compares each practice to a mini-company, with
all of the companies aligned around *The BAYADA Way*.

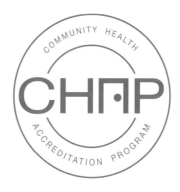

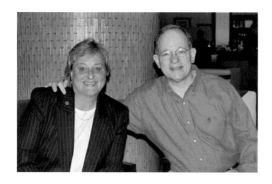

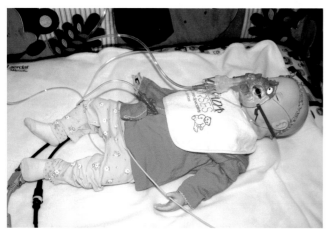

ABOVE: BAYADA proudly displayed
the CHAP logo on its materials after
becoming accredited in 2008.

LEFT: The work of Anne Johnson,
Division Director of Policy
Development, was vital to the
CHAP process. She is shown with
Mark at the 2008 Awards Weekend.

BELOW: An interactive baby
manikin. BAYADA's pediatric
simulation program for home care is
the first of its kind in the country.

Major steps forward

Affirmation of BAYADA's excellence reached a new level
with its 2008 Community Health Accreditation Program
(CHAP) accreditation, which assures clients and referral
sources that BAYADA meets the industry's highest quality
standards in its home care operations.

The investments in education and alignment throughout the decade had an unexpected benefit. They helped
BAYADA weather the severe recession that began in 2008
exceptionally well. The company was also able to establish
a Hospice Specialty Practice, which has doubled in size
since its start in 2009. "It's just amazing to be part of an
organization that quarter after quarter has grown," says
Karen Hojda, Director of Leadership Development and Talent
Management in Burlington, New Jersey. Having worked at
a publicly held company, Karen knows the upheavals that
recessions can cause. "We feel like we're in 'The BAYADA
Bubble' because we keep growing—we're hiring when
other companies aren't," she adds.

Also as part of the new millennium, BAYADA training
programs continued to take advantage of advances in
technology. High-tech simulation training enhances field
employees' skills by simulating real-life and real-time
scenarios, preparing them to handle emergencies. BAYADA
employees developed the scenarios, policies, and evaluation tools that are specific to home care in order to prepare
nurses to care for clients with complex needs in the comfort
of their own homes. Charlotte, North Carolina, is home
to the company's first adult simulation lab where home
care professionals can get firsthand, hands-on experience.

Supporting each other

The BAYADA Way is not just a guiding force at work. It's often the inspiration for how employees live, both in happy times and sadder ones.

Bethany Preston, a Nurse Clinical Manager who had been battling cervical cancer, learned in January 2013 that her condition was terminal. Upon hearing this news, Mark and Ann Baiada made a special trip to visit Bethany at her home in Shelby, North Carolina.

Not knowing they were coming, Bethany was shocked to see them.

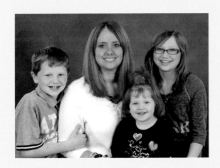

"I can't believe Mark Baiada is in my bedroom!" she exclaimed, brightening the mood far beyond expectations. Bethany's older children were in on the secret but hadn't given it away. Several of Bethany's colleagues were on hand, including Joe Seidel, who organized the logistics, and Melinda Phillips, then a Regional Director. Bethany was presented with a plaque of appreciation and a bouquet of flowers. Marie Blessington's office and division further honored Bethany with a very moving Ann Baiada Award nomination.

The visit's intent was to follow *The BAYADA Way* by "showing love" in a tangible way. Bethany felt loved and appreciated. She commented that the support she and her family received from BAYADA throughout her illness taught her much about life and how to treat others.

Bethany passed away four months later. Her radiance and courage live on in the memories of her husband John, their children Brayden (age 12), Trevor (age 10), and Kadence (age 3), and her BAYADA coworkers and clients. ✿

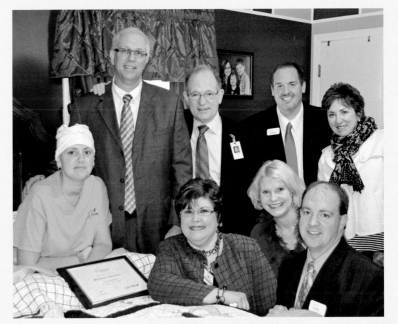

BELOW LEFT: Bethany and her children.

BELOW: BAYADA colleagues on the visit to Bethany's home. Back row: Clinical Manager Bethany Preston, Division Director Joe Seidel, Mark, CSM Mark Bowling, and Ann. Front row: Clinical Manager Marsha Armstrong, ASPIRE Nurse Anna-Lena Stone, and CSM Jack Hight.

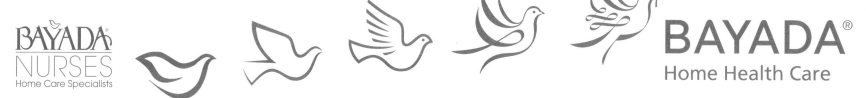

Additionally, BAYADA's pediatric simulation program, involving an interactive baby manikin, is the first of its kind for pediatric home care in the country. Kim Lynn, Clinical Support Specialist in Clinical Standards and Quality, designed the initial scenarios and protocols. Sadly, Kim was killed in an automobile accident in August 2012. A total of 24 pediatric simulation labs located in Pennsylvania, New Jersey, New York, Massachusetts, North Carolina, and Georgia are dedicated to her memory.

The company's momentum continued with a huge rebranding effort. The name "BAYADA Nurses" had not fully encompassed the company's services for decades, and alignment underscored the urgent need for a more inclusive name. BAYADA Home Health Care was the logical choice.

The logo and related design elements needed to change with the times, too. A dove had symbolized BAYADA Nurses, chosen as an icon of peace and love. Keeping it was non-negotiable, but updating it was not an easy feat, as Janice Lovequist recalls. She helped manage the process with an outside firm while working as a company graphic designer. (Janice has since become Manager of *The BAYADA Way* Team.) In keeping with the desire for consensus, surveys ensued. "Mark wants to vet everything and make sure everybody's happy, so we had multiple options," says Janice. "People usually don't like change, though, and everyone was picking the logos with our old dove." The group ultimately settled on an elegantly restyled dove that now feels as familiar as the previous one had.

Ongoing commitment to community service

Beyond direct client care, giving back to the community is part of what BAYADA stands for. In addition to the company's unstinting sponsorship of the BAYADA Regatta—the longest running adaptive rowing competition for people with disabilities—"doing good" takes the form of countless charitable acts.

Individual employees and entire offices regularly serve causes of their choosing, often to support local efforts or honor a BAYADA employee or client. Clothing donations for the Salvation Army, fun-runs for disease research, roll-up-your-sleeves help during disasters such as Hurricane Sandy—whatever the cause, BAYADA people come through.

Many efforts combine fun and service. At a recognition picnic for field employees and their families in 2013, the Willow Grove, Pennsylvania, assistive care office raised money for a client, Abi, who had suffered traumatic brain injury after a car accident. She required nursing care 16 hours a day. Collecting through raffle baskets, the office raised money for a nonprofit foundation that supported her cause.

Here is another example of giving back on a more personal scale: In 2014, the Vermont Rutland Hospice office hosted its first memorial picnic and service for families of clients who had passed away. The attendees created colorful prayer flags, recited poems, and tossed rose petals in a pond—activities that celebrated the lives of their loved ones and aided in their own recovery from grief.

ABOVE: Metamorphosis of the logo and dove took years and involved many discussions, surveys, and outside design consultants. The three doves shown in the middle were options that were never used.

OPPOSITE TOP TO BOTTOM: University City (Philadelphia) employees cooked for a local charity.

Suzanne Collins, Clinical Associate, presents a donation from the Delaware Pediatric offices to the Ronald McDonald House of Delaware.

Employees from the Williamsport Adult and Lewisburg Adult assistive care state programs offices in Pennsylvania at a Walk to End Alzheimer's.

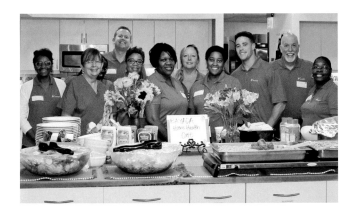

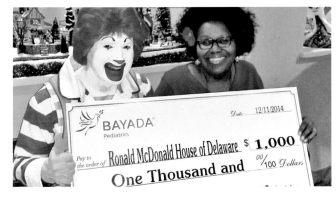

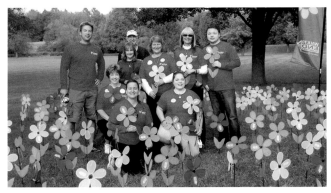

The gift of the Moravian star

Sometimes the simplest gifts in life are the most powerful. As a kind gesture, longtime client Lynn W. sent Mark Baiada one of her handmade Moravian-style paper star ornaments at Christmas 2011. Impressed with its complexity and purity, Mark thought it would make a great gift for the BAYADA offices. So he asked Lynn to make a star for each of the 350 offices for the next Christmas.

Lynn was flattered. In July 2012, she started constructing the stars, which involved cutting and intricately folding four strips of paper for each one. A total of 1,400 cut strips of paper and many hours of work later, the stars were completed. She sent them to Headquarters employees, who affixed a message from Mark and distributed them to all offices.

Lynn, who had spina bifida and used a ventilator, performed the work even though she required around-the-clock care from BAYADA's Winston-Salem, North Carolina, adult nursing office. Her smile and optimism were infectious, according to those who knew her.

In December of that year, Lynn became sick and was hospitalized. Mark called Lynn that Christmas Eve at the hospital. He thanked her for her meaningful gift to the offices and wished her a happy holiday. Lynn's parents said she was very touched by his call.

Sadly, Lynn passed away two days later, but her memory and her Moravian stars live on. In fact, Mark still has his star in his office at Headquarters and cherishes it. 🌿

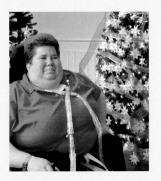

Client Lynn W. proudly displayed her handmade stars in Winston-Salem, North Carolina, shortly before her passing in 2012.

BAYADA client Lynn, so graciously handmade over 300 of these modest stars, which remind us that the smallest and most simple things in life are just as precious. Happy Holidays – Mark Baiada

"Millions of people worldwide"

BAYADA's financial strength enabled it to acquire Nursefinders Home Care in 2012. This added 16 offices nationwide and gave BAYADA its first lasting presence across an ocean, albeit in the state of Hawaii. In 2013, the company partnered with India Home Health Care (IHHC), which serves the major cities of Chennai and Bangalore. "They'd been around for a few years, and they were looking for an additional investor and expertise," says Mark. BAYADA is helping the IHHC team increase its business and expand geographically. The partnership may result in European growth as well. Frank Goller, IHHC's

founding president and a native of Germany, is helping BAYADA actively seek opportunities to provide home health care in Germany.

At home in the U.S., BAYADA hopes to align with hospital health systems as the preferred provider, exclusively managing their home health services. "That's our expertise," Mark emphasizes, "recruiting, training, and developing a compassionate, excellent, reliable work force to do home health care." Expansion of a different sort is also happening at BAYADA's long-time Headquarters location in Moorestown, New Jersey. After renting 290 Chester Avenue for 33 years, the company

BELOW RIGHT: The new Headquarters building in Moorestown.

BELOW: Mark and Mel Baiada received a warm welcome from India Home Health Care colleagues in 2015. The brothers traveled to Chennai, where Mark chaired a conference panel on the Evolution of Home Health Care in India.

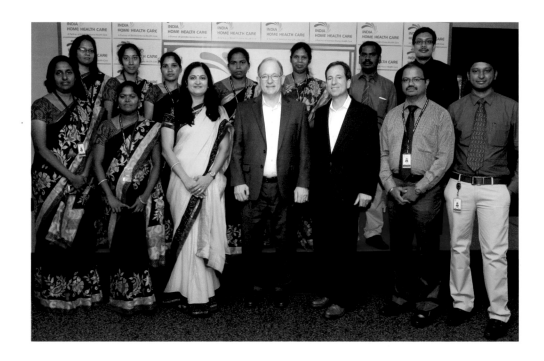

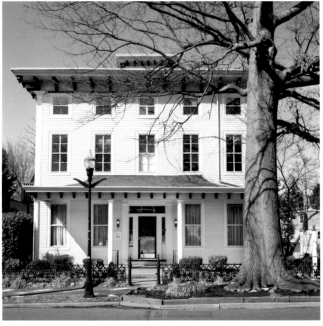

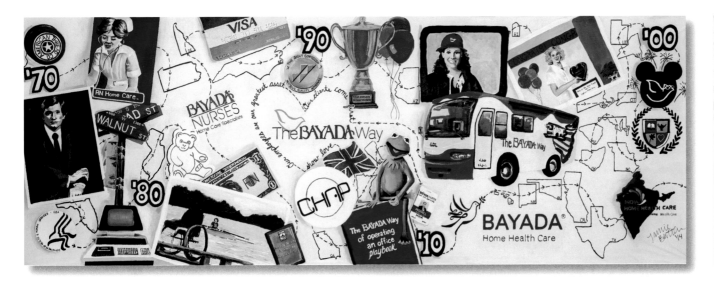

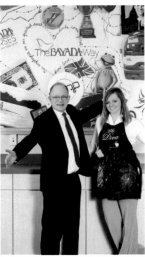

purchased a historic building nearby. Headquarters employees will move into 1 West Main Street in 2015, a fitting transition for the fortieth anniversary year.

And the company's history literally went on display at its New Jersey Learning Center in the form of a colorful 14-foot mural by Jamie Buttler, a member of the Communication (COM) office's internal team. Jamie is a multi-talented woman whose credentials include a Master's Degree in Art Therapy. The whole world can view the mural, thanks to a 44-second Facebook and YouTube time-lapse video that captures the 27 hours it took Jamie to paint it!

As BAYADA Home Health Care moves into its fifth decade, employees from all eras can take deep pride in what they have created: an international company with

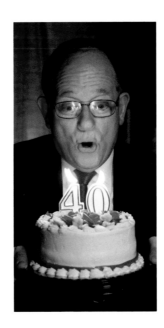

290 service offices across 21 states in the U.S. and a presence in India, with some 23,000 employees serving 26,000 clients and families. Mark hopes that in 100 years, BAYADA will be the world's most trusted team of health care professionals, with hundreds of thousands of employees serving millions of people worldwide.

ABOVE: Mark and Jamie Buttler at the mural unveiling. Jamie's Artist's Statement concludes with these inspiring words: "I hope this mural serves as an enduring tribute to the vision of Mark Baiada and how, together, we have all played a role in shaping the first 40 years of BAYADA."

LEFT: Mark on January 17, 2015, exactly 40 years after his company was incorporated.

Acres of Diamonds

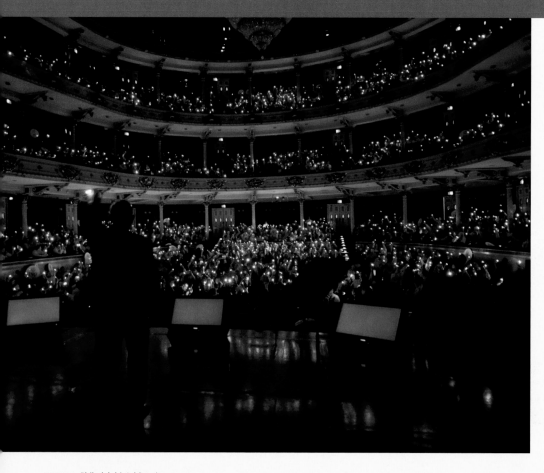

ABOVE: Philadelphia's historic Academy of Music glowed with the lights and love of 2,000 employees at the 2011 Awards Weekend.

RIGHT: A twist of the "diamond" lit up each employee's ring.

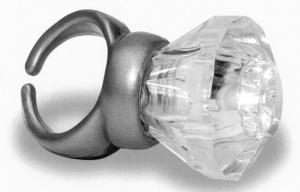

"Absolutely incredible. It sent a message that will last a lifetime."

"I still get goose bumps when I think of all those diamond rings lighting up the darkness. It was so awesome that it brought me to tears. What a magnificent sight! I will never forget it."

"It really demonstrated the growth of the company and how we all play a part in making it shine."

"As I listened to Mark tell the story of the diamonds, I truly felt as a valued part of something far greater than myself! Little by little, as the diamonds were lit, then the whole room was bright with the lights of all the BAYADA team, it truly displayed how as a team, we can light the whole world! THANK YOU!"

Mark Baiada has a deep talent for making people feel special. At the 2011 Awards Weekend in Philadelphia, he made employees collectively shine brighter than ever. Upon entering the beautiful and historic Academy of Music grand opera house, each employee received an LED "diamond" ring. Then, Mark held the audience of 2,000 spellbound as he told a tale about "Acres of Diamonds."

The tale concerns a Persian, Ali Hafed by name, who sells his house and relentlessly searches the world for diamonds to make him rich. He grows poor and dies in the process. What he never realized was that acres of diamonds were in his own backyard garden all along—the garden he had sold.

This parable was first set down in English by Russell Conwell, the founder and first president of Temple

University, who heard it as a traveler in the Middle East in 1869. Reverend Conwell used it as the basis of a lecture that he delivered 6,000 times, and it's the reason Temple's football team still wears diamond decals on their helmets and diamond trim on their collars. Mark loves the story and connected it to his own experience, telling BAYADA employees that "I see diamonds in all of you." Here is part of his talk that night:

We are in constant search for a better way, but like Ali Hafed, we may be looking for it in the wrong places. We may be better served if we look inward, to see what is in us to capitalize on.

I, too, have had temptations, like Ali Hafed. I, too, have had moments where I have been distracted, or even tempted, to go for that one big diamond. There have been times where I was approached to sell the company, or go public. They promised me a huge diamond. . . . Yet, I had another moment of truth—that the diamond they were offering was limited, because they would take me far away from where there were many more diamonds than I could ever imagine. I realized that I am a person who is motivated by a much bigger picture, much bigger than one big diamond and selling out.

I am motivated by caring for millions of people worldwide in the comfort of their own home. I am motivated by the fact that my acres of diamonds are right in front of me. Let me tell you why I say that, and what I see, when I look at you. I see diamonds in all of you. Yes, they're there. Some may need polishing, and some may be in the rough, but I do see them.

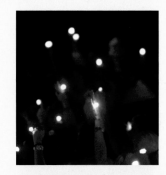

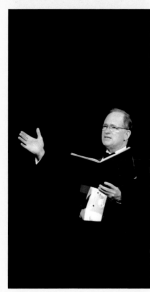

TOP: Upraised hands set the theater aglow.

ABOVE: "I am motivated by the fact that my acres of diamonds are right in front of me."

Just imagine when we cultivate our own diamonds, how bright, happy, and more successful we will become. Even greater, imagine if we cultivate the diamonds that are in our offices, the diamonds inside the people in the field. It will help us achieve our vision faster of serving millions of people worldwide in the comfort of their own homes.

Next, to illustrate "the power of working together," Mark asked for all of the lights to be turned off. The theater went black, sending shivers up everyone's spines. Then, he lit his own diamond ring. "Can you see it? Just one little diamond," Mark said. Those eight words, spoken softly into the darkness, are still making waves. Next, he asked all the employees from the 1970s to light their rings, followed by those from the 1980s and the 1990s. Finally those from the 2000s—the majority of employees—lit their rings, setting the theater dramatically aglow.

"This came out a lot better than I thought it would," Mark joked. But his eyes were filled with tears, as were most everyone else's.

Marie Blessington, RN, who was backstage, saw the scene from Mark's viewpoint. "The view I had was so incredible. Once all the rings were lit, all you could see was a sea of diamonds. It was amazing. That picture will never leave my mind," says Marie. "It was definitely a 'wow' moment."

Patty Watson, RN, still revels in the memory. "Mark told all of us we were his gems," says Patty, a Division Director in New Castle, Delaware. "What a brilliant way to make us feel so special!" ❦

BAYADA Milestones

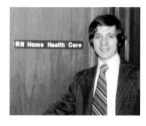

RN Home Care.

1973
Having long planned to start a business, J. Mark Baiada commits to researching business opportunities with the hopes of starting a company within the next few years.

1975
RN Home Health Care, Inc., is incorporated on January 17 at 1426 Walnut Street in Philadelphia.

1978
RN Home Health Care opens its second service office, in Florida.

1980
RN Home Health Care's Philadelphia office receives the company's first Medicare certification.

1983
The BAYADA Regatta takes place on the banks of the Schuylkill River in Philadelphia, where the all-adaptive rowing event is still held today.

1989
BAYADA Nurses hires its first rehabilitation nurse, Ann Claffey, RN, CRRN, and adds rehabilitation nursing services to its offerings.

1993
BAYADA Nurses earns accreditation with commendation from the Joint Commission on the Accreditation of Health Care Organizations (JCAHO).

| 1975 | 1976 | 1977 | 1978 | 1979 | 1980 | 1981 | 1982 | 1983 | 1984 | 1985 | 1986 | 1987 | 1988 | 1989 | 1990 | 1991 | 1992 | 1993 | 1994 | 1995 |

1 Service Office

11 Service Offices

24 Service Offices

1976
The Philadelphia Corporation for Aging™ (PCA) awards the company a contract that doubles its business.

1977
The company invests in its first computer for payroll and billing.

1979
The Muppet Movie and its character Kermit the Frog make a profound impact on Mark.

1982
RN Home Health Care has expanded to six offices in Pennsylvania, New Jersey, Florida, and Colorado. It moves its headquarters to Moorestown, New Jersey.

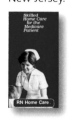

1983
The company changes its name to BAYADA Nurses both to differentiate itself in a growing market and to personalize the company name. Mark uses the phonetic spelling of his last name because Baiada is more difficult to spell and pronounce.

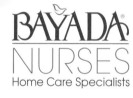

1991
Mark and Ann Claffey are married. Their blended family includes Mark's children, David and Janice, and Ann's daughters Jaclyn, Kelli, and Christin.

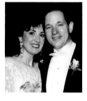

1995
Reflecting major changes in the U.S. health care landscape, the company opens a Managed Care office to receive referrals and manage care for regional and national payors.

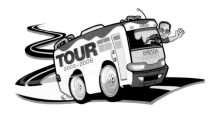
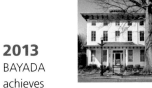

1998
A heart-warming television commercial entitled "Heroes on the Home Front" airs in key markets.

2000
BAYADA Nurses celebrates its 25th anniversary in Disney World at the company's annual Awards Weekend.

2000s
Employee education opportunities, ranging from Presidential Scholarships to webinars, evolve and grow as part of BAYADA University.

2005–2006
The BAYADA Way document debuts. To share the spirit across the company, Mark and Ann Baiada launch *The BAYADA Way* Bus Tour, an eight-month road trip to visit all 124 offices in 15 states.

2008–2010
Alignment begins, culminating in the creation of eight specialty practices: Home Health, Adult Nursing, Assistive Care, Assistive Care State Programs, Pediatrics, Habilitation, Hospice, and Staffing.

2013
BAYADA achieves its dream of being international through a strategic partnership with India Home Health Care.

2015
BAYADA moves its headquarters to a historic home on Main Street in Moorestown, New Jersey.

1996 1997 1998 1999 2000 2001 2002 2003 2004 2005 2006 2007 2008 2009 2010 2011 2012 2013 2014 2015 . . . .

101 Service Offices

290 Service Offices

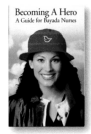

1999
The "Hero on the Home Front" employee recognition program begins (later renamed the Hero Program).

2002
Al Freedman, PhD, a psychologist and the father of Jack, a medically fragile BAYADA pediatric client, joins Mark in a three-year process to define the company's mission, vision, values, and beliefs.

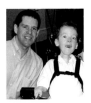

2008
The BAYADA Way of Operating an Office rolls out, putting professional standards of practice into place to align service offices with *The BAYADA Way*.

The company is accredited by the Community Health Accreditation Program (CHAP).

2012
BAYADA Nurses is changed to BAYADA Home Health Care to more clearly and consistently communicate BAYADA's breadth of services, its team of multi-disciplinary professionals, and its dedication to *The BAYADA Way*.

2015
At its 40th anniversary, BAYADA employs almost 3,000 office employees and more than 20,000 home health care professionals who provide care to 26,000 clients per week from 290 offices in 21 states and India.

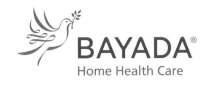

Recognize and Reward: "Our Employees Are Our Greatest Asset"

From everyday exchanges between coworkers to expressions of gratitude from clients, a culture of appreciation and recognition permeates BAYADA. It started the day the company opened for business and has been nurtured ever since.

Preserving and sharing those expressions of gratitude are central to BAYADA's way of working. From the earliest company newsletters onward to the *BAYADA Bulletin*, issues have included thank-you notes from clients and their families, as well as notes of gratitude from company leaders.

And when offices meet goals and otherwise do an outstanding job, the company sends tangible thanks in the form of gift cards, candy, flowers, and other mementos. "It's so easy just to say thank you, and it really makes a difference," says Anita Palmer, Project Coordinator, who manages the process of sending billing record gifts. The feelings flow both ways. Mark and Ann cherish notes of gratitude from employees.

The company also highlights certain aspects of *The BAYADA Way* for an entire year through campaigns such as the Year of Gratitude, Year of Recognition, and Year of Reliability, providing tools and resources to promote and celebrate the theme. Parties, awards, and recognition are an integral part of the campaigns—carrying forward the "work hard, play hard" ethic that has characterized BAYADA since the beginning.

As *The BAYADA Way* states succinctly: "We believe our employees are our greatest asset." When you have a valuable asset, you protect it, and the company does just that through the following recognition programs and awards.

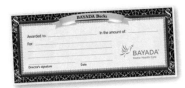

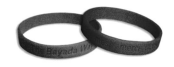

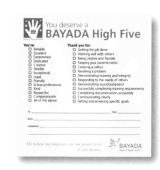

TOP TO BOTTOM: BAYADA Bucks can be earned and redeemed in a number of ways.

Year of Gratitude bracelets are given in sets of two—one to keep and one to give as a thank-you.

High Five notepads make it easy to compliment coworkers.

Year of Reliability pledge cards helped employees live up to self-made promises.

Recognition Programs

BAYADA Bucks

Recipients may earn BAYADA Bucks by attaining perfect attendance, covering last-minute callouts, being named the employee of the month, and more. As their BAYADA Bucks accrue, employees can spend them on branded merchandise, items for everyday use, or even high-end gifts in the BAYADA Bucks Catalog.

BAYADA High Five

As part of the Year of Recognition, the BAYADA High Five evolved into an ongoing program that encourages daily recognition for coworkers and colleagues. Materials that depict a hand giving a high-five carry the personally written messages on buttons, stickers, greeting cards, postcards, and notepads.

Years of Service

Through the Years of Service program, BAYADA recognizes attributes such as loyalty and commitment. Tenured field employees are awarded with certificates, special awards or gifts, and specific BAYADA Bucks denominations, which they may redeem for a gift of their choice. Office employees honorees receive their awards at the annual Awards Weekend celebration. At the 2015 event, more than 240 office employees were recognized for service ranging from five to 40 years.

Companywide Contests

Annual, companywide field employee contests are designed around a specific theme supporting *The BAYADA Way.* The contests are promoted through communications, office decorations, and weekly prizes to honor and recognize all employees who demonstrate company values.

Recognition Awards

To inspire employees and reward those who go above and beyond in different areas of client care, BAYADA regularly presents special recognition awards. Candidates are nominated by their peers.

The Ann Baiada Award for Clinical Excellence

An inspiring leader and a true nurse's nurse, Ann Baiada, RN, CRRN, has made countless contributions to BAYADA since she started in 1989. One of her crowning achievements is the BAYADAbility program, established in 1998. This unique, enhanced rehabilitation nursing care program has helped set the company apart.

"Ann is a personal hero of mine," says Marie Blessington, RN, Director of Clinical Leadership Development at the Clinical Standards and Quality office in Moorestown, New Jersey. To continue Ann's legacy of empowering, inspiring, and supporting others, Marie initiated The Ann Baiada Award for Clinical Excellence in 2006, with Ann as its first recipient. A committee chooses an outstanding clinical leader each year and bestows the honor at Awards Weekend.

The Linda Siessel Award for Excellence in Client Services Leadership

To honor Linda Siessel's outstanding contributions to BAYADA client services, the company created an award in her honor. "I received a surprise of a lifetime, the first award for Client Services Leadership," says Linda, Home Care Chief Operating Officer. "To have it named after me was unbelievable. I was deeply humbled to be acknowledged

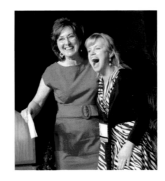

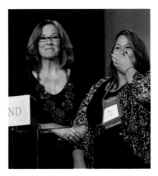

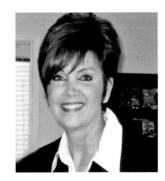

TOP TO BOTTOM: Ann and Susan Ecker Sterner receiving the Ann Baiada Award in 2008.

Linda and Tara Robinson receiving the Linda Siessel Award in 2012.

Pat Mallee's inspiration lives on.

in this way. The best part is now being able to present this award to fellow colleagues, and to see them shine and be celebrated by their families, friends, and co-workers." A committee chooses an outstanding Client Services leader each year and bestows the honor at Awards Weekend.

The subsequent recipient, Anna Anderson, spent the first 10 years of her career working for Linda, whom she deeply admires. "There are no words to describe what it was really like, being on stage with 3,000 people in the audience watching me receive it," says Anna, who is Client Services Manager in the assistive care office in Morristown, New Jersey. "The energy and excitement was high. It was the proudest moment of my whole life."

The Pat Mallee Award for Compassionate Leadership

Known as an "enormously compassionate" and "amazing" nurse, leader, friend, and champion, Pat Mallee, Regional Director of the Shamrock Group (Skilled Visit Services), passed away in 2011 after a battle with cancer. In her years at BAYADA, she gained widespread respect for her clinical knowledge, positive spirit, and professionalism.

"There was no person who was more committed to the growth and success of Medicare-certified home health services at BAYADA than Pat," says David Baiada, Chief Operating Officer, Home Health, Hospice, and Quality. "She brought expertise, energy, conviction, and passion. Pat's vision, unwavering positive spirit, and commitment to *The BAYADA Way* are an inspiration to all who knew her." To honor role models like Pat, the company established the annual Pat Mallee Award for Compassionate Leadership.

Hero Program

Inspired by BAYADA's Heroes on the Home Front television campaign, the BAYADA Hero Program is one of many programs devoted to recognizing and rewarding home health care professionals who consistently demonstrate the core values of *The BAYADA Way.* "Their work epitomizes our mission of helping people have a safe home life with comfort, independence, and dignity by providing the highest quality home health care services available," says Mark Baiada. Office employees and clients can nominate any registered nurse, licensed practical nurse, home health aide, or other professional caregivers. Heroes are recognized at the office, division, and national level.

Hero Program awards are the high point of the annual Awards Weekends. National honorees, with their families and sometimes their clients in attendance, receive ovations from their peers. Their work is commemorated in videos that debut at the event and are showcased on the company's website and on YouTube.

The Hero Program also includes three awards that have been earned by hundreds of dedicated individuals and teams. The Lifesaver Hero Award acknowledges individuals who perform extraordinary or lifesaving deeds. The Team Spirit Hero Award recognizes groups of health care professionals whose team efforts make it possible for clients to remain at home. The Remarkable Rookie Hero Award salutes newer employees who are shining stars.

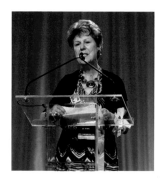

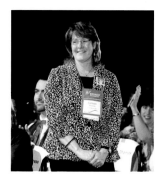

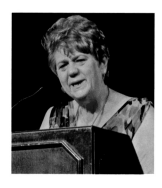

TOP TO BOTTOM: Anna Anderson thanking colleagues for the Linda Siessel Award in 2012.

Colleen Thomas being recognized as the 2012 Pat Mallee Award honoree.

Cathy Akbari, the 2011 Registered Nurse National Hero.

Recognition Program Awardees

The Ann Baiada Award for Clinical Excellence

2006
Ann Baiada
Director
Moorestown, NJ
HQ—Headquarters

2008
Susan Ecker Sterner
Senior RN, Transitional Care Manager
Philadelphia, PA
SWP—Sweet Pea pediatric division

2009
Patricia Pagano
Clinical Manager
Langhorne, PA
LBA—Assistive care

2010
Emma Garvin
Clinical Manager
Eden, NC
EDE—Assistive care state programs

2011
Cecilia Weber
Clinical Manager
King of Prussia, PA
KOP—Assistive care state programs

2012
Kathryn Hawley
Pediatric Clinical Operations Manager
Winston-Salem, NC
FRS—Freesia pediatric division

2013
Teresa Lee
Clinical Educator
York, PA
YRK—Pediatrics

2014
Amy Doerrman
Associate Director
Reading, PA
REA—Pediatrics

2014
Karen "Myke" McKinney
Associate Director
Charlotte, NC
CPC—Assistive care

The Linda Siessel Award for Excellence in Client Services Leadership

2012
Linda Siessel
Chief Operating Officer
Morristown, NJ
HCS—Home Care Services support office

2013
Anna Anderson
Client Services Manager
Morristown, NJ
MOR—Assistive care

2014
Tara Robinson
Client Services Manager
Wilmington, DE
DSP—Assistive care state programs

The Pat Mallee Award for Compassionate Leadership

2012

Colleen Thomas
Area Director
Langhorne, PA
IS—Information Services support office

2013

Dawn King
Area Director
Blue Bell, PA
MCV—Home health

2014

Cindy Istvan
Director
Burlington, NJ
PRC—Pediatric Regulatory Compliance support office

National Heroes of the Year

2000

Elsie Hartigan
Licensed Practical Nurse
Burlington, NJ
BP—Pediatrics

Betsy Earnhardt
Registered Nurse
Winston-Salem, NC
WS—Former pediatric and adult nursing service office

Ina Howell
Home Health Aide
Pinellas Park, FL
PP—Former full service office

2001

Iris Rodriguez
Home Health Aide
Philadelphia, PA
PCA—Assistive care state programs

Charles Costello
Licensed Practical Nurse
Burlington, NJ
BUR—Assistive care

Nancy Bojarski
Registered Nurse
Burlington, NJ
BUR—Assistive care

2002

Margaret Galletto
Certified Home Health Aide
Morristown, NJ
MOR—Assistive care

Gwen Ingram
Licensed Practical Nurse
Lawrenceville, NJ
LAW—Former full service office

Gloria Lindsay
Registered Nurse
Wilmington, DE
WIL—Home health

2003

Rose Lewis
Home Health Aide
Philadelphia, PA
PCA—Assistive care state programs

Barbara Mizialko
Licensed Practical Nurse
Willow Grove, PA
WG—Assistive care

Linda Wall
Registered Nurse
Charlotte, NC
CHA—Adult nursing

2004

Maria L. Garcia
Home Health Aide
Union, NJ
UNI—Assistive care state programs

Maryann Parvesse
Licensed Practical Nurse
Lawrenceville, NJ
LAW—Former full service office

Lee Stengel
Registered Nurse
Burlington, NJ
BUR—Assistive care

2005

Sallie Lipps
Home Health Aide
Winston-Salem, NC
WSA—Adult nursing

Katherine Cashier
Licensed Practical Nurse
Greensboro, NC
GRE—Adult nursing

Joan Church
Registered Nurse
Winston-Salem, NC
WSA—Adult nursing

2006

Uriel Worthington
Home Health Aide
Philadelphia, PA
PCA—Assistive care state programs

Kim Stewart
Licensed Practical Nurse
New Castle, DE
DP—Pediatrics

Sharon Grecco
Registered Nurse
Voorhees, NJ
VP—Pediatrics

2007

Helena Miller
Home Health Aide
Wilmington, DE
WPD—Former adult nursing and assistive care service office

Deborah McIntyre
Licensed Practical Nurse
Lawrenceville, NJ
LAW—Former full service office

Barry Finnigan
Registered Nurse
Charlotte, NC
CHA—Adult nursing

2008

Anita Boehme
Physical Therapist
Tucson, AZ
TWV—Home health

Connie Smith
Home Health Aide
Willow Grove, PA
WG—Assistive care

Shirley Hedin
Licensed Practical Nurse
Toms River, NJ
TR—Assistive care state programs

Caroll Maholick
Registered Nurse
Charlotte, NC
CHA—Adult nursing

2009

Steven Conforti
Physical Therapist
Phoenix, AZ
PHO—Home health

Stephanie Hill
Home Health Aide
North Brunswick, NJ
NB—Assistive care

George Kracke
Licensed Practical Nurse
North Brunswick, NJ
NBP—Pediatrics

Marjorie Smith-Gale
Registered Nurse
Linwood, NJ
AC—Adult nursing

2010

Joan Beroth
Medical Social Worker
Tucson, AZ
TEV—Home health

Ray Woods
Licensed Practical Nurse
Charlotte, NC
CHA—Adult nursing

Brett Miller
Registered Nurse
Minnetonka, MN
MNP—Pediatrics

2011

Barbara Sauer
Medical Social Worker
Denver, CO
DV—Home health

Jane Harrison
Home Health Aide
Main Line, PA
MLA—Assistive care

Toni Kearns
Licensed Practical Nurse
Lewisburg, PA
LEW—Assistive care state programs

Cathy Akbari
Registered Nurse
Charlotte, NC
CHP—Pediatrics

2012

John Robinson
Physical Therapist
Upper Bucks, PA
UBV—Home health

Maria Ortega de Rivera
Certified Nursing Assistant
Tampa, FL
TAM—Assistive care

Lorraine McMillan
Licensed Practical Nurse
Reading, PA
REA—Pediatrics

Deirdre Dutka
Registered Nurse
King of Prussia, PA
KOP—Assistive care state programs

2013

John Morris
Registered Nurse
Charlotte, NC
CHA—Adult nursing

Amber Lehman
Licensed Practical Nurse
Williamsport, PA
WLM—Pediatrics

Leonard Barringer
Certified Occupational Therapy Assistant
Cabarrus, NC
CAV—Home health

Judy Morrison
Home Health Aide
Harrisburg, PA
HAR—Assistive care state programs

2014

Sherri Lorette
Registered Nurse
Norwich, Vermont
VTH—Hospice

Kevin Shreckengast
Licensed Practical Nurse
Williamsport, PA
WLM—Pediatrics

Karen Richards-Monaghan
Physical Therapist
Delaware County, PA
DCF—Home health

Regina Derby
Certified Home Health Aide
Atlantic City, NJ
AC—Adult nursing

2015

David Hill
Physical Therapist
Cabarrus County, NC
CAV—Home health

Tracey Read
Certified Nursing Assistant
Shelby, NC
SHE—Assistive care state programs

David Birnbaum
Licensed Practical Nurse
East Stroudsburg, PA
ESP—Pediatrics

Kenneth Gebhardt
Registered Nurse
Downingtown, PA
DOW—Pediatrics

Acknowledgments

It has been a fantastic ride for me researching, interviewing, and writing the BAYADA 40-year history book. Never before have I worked with such a large group of similarly professional, reliable, and truly kind people who have so much in common: wanting to do good and help others.

I got to see firsthand *The BAYADA Way* played out in a variety of situations. One of my favorite parts of research was attending home visits with Ellen Wiest, RN, CRRN. She's a hardworking, energetic Clinical Manager with a great sense of humor. Ellen introduced me to a few clients she supervises. One of her longtime clients, Tony, who has been living with quadriplegia for two decades, relies on nurses all days of the week except one when family steps in. Ellen and Tony helped open my eyes to what it's really like to live with a catastrophic, chronic condition, but even more so to how reliant Tony is on receiving excellent care to keep him out of hospitals. I also saw his long-term, regular nurse, Debbie, working with him. It's no wonder Tony loves his BAYADA nurses!

In writing this book, I interviewed dozens of employees (both current and retired) and family members. I'd like to thank each one of them for their time and assistance. Most important were Mark Baiada and Ann Baiada. The other extremely helpful and enthusiastic interviewees included Anna Anderson, David Baiada, Mel Baiada, Marie Blessington, Bruce Bosco, Marty (Bodor) Boughey, Melissa Burnside, Karen Buttler, Barbara Colin, Marion Fiero, Al Freedman, Andrew Gentile, Ginny Gotides, Christin Gregory, Maureen Hixon, Karen Hojda, Werner Hoppe, Anne Johnson, Jackie

Kirchhoff, Bonnie Carr Long, Janice Lovequist, Debra Magaraci, Kelli Marans, Carole McMahon, Peggy Morrison, Jean Mullin, Tom Mylet, Hilary Osborne, Anita Palmer, Melinda Phillips, Sherri Pillet, Kathy Reavy, Karen Rizzo, Ann Schaller, Tom Sibson, Linda Siessel, Marty Soroka, Susie Ecker Sterner, Colleen Thomas, Cris Toscano, David Totaro, Laurel Trice, Sharon Vogel, Patty Watson, Holly White, Ellen Wiest, Joanne Wilson, and Maureen Wright.

This book could not have been possible without the undying and always timely assistance of Headquarters staff members Janice Lovequist and Stephanie Smith, as well as Hilary Osborne and her team in the Communications Office. You all helped in more ways than you can imagine. Overall, I'd like to thank the entire BAYADA family for their warm, welcoming, and helpful nature as well as their collective sense of humor. It makes writing a book even more fulfilling when everyone is so willing to help tell fabulous stories—both happy and sad.

Thanks also to my project manager/editor, Marian Calabro, who has been a great partner, always striving for excellence. And to art director Chris Reynolds for designing a truly beautiful book. Final thanks go to my own family for their support and sacrifice in helping me complete this book: Bill, Joey, Tommy, and Will (and our loveable dog, Harry). You guys are what inspire me daily.

Working on this book caused me to regularly reflect on what the field staff endures to make sure their clients are cared for with kindness, dignity, and respect. To them, I dedicate this book.

—*Christine McLaughlin*

About the Creative Team

Christine McLaughlin, Author. Christine writes and edits nonfiction articles and books on a variety of topics for private and nonprofit clients. She's the author of *The Dog Lover's Companion to Philadelphia* and *Philadelphia: A Photographic Portrait.* Christine is also the coauthor of *American Red Cross: Dog First Aid* and *American Red Cross: Cat First Aid.* Her health care clients have included Abington Memorial Hospital, ADVANCE for Nurses, ADVANCE for Physical Therapists & PT Assistants, Einstein Healthcare Network, and Fox Chase Cancer Center. Christine lives in Oreland, Pennsylvania.

Marian Calabro, Editor and Project Manager. As the president of CorporateHistory.net, Marian directs business anniversary projects for clients across the United States. She has also written corporate history books for The Clorox Company, Public Service Electric & Gas, The Pep Boys—Manny, Moe & Jack, and many others. Marian is based in Hasbrouck Heights, New Jersey.

Christine Reynolds, Production Manager and Art Director. Christine specializes in historical publications and exhibitions. In addition to business histories designed for CorporateHistory.net, she has produced anniversary books for Brown Brothers Harriman, the YMCA of Greater Boston, and divisions of Harvard University. Christine is based in Waltham, Massachusetts.

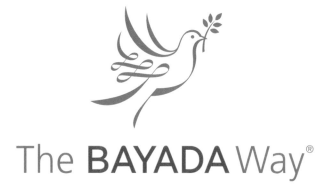

The **BAYADA** Way®

Our Mission

BAYADA Home Health Care has a special purpose—to help people have a safe home life with comfort, independence, and dignity. BAYADA Home Health Care provides nursing, rehabilitative, therapeutic, hospice, and assistive care services to children, adults, and seniors worldwide. We care for our clients 24 hours a day, 7 days a week.

Families coping with significant illness or disability need help and support while caring for a family member. Our goal at BAYADA is to provide the highest quality home health care services available. We believe our clients and their families deserve home health care delivered with **compassion, excellence,** and **reliability,** our BAYADA core values.

Our Vision

With a strong commitment from each of us, BAYADA Home Health Care will make it possible for millions of people worldwide to experience a better quality of life in the comfort of their own homes. We want to build and maintain a lasting legacy as the world's most compassionate and trusted team of home health care professionals.

We will accomplish our mission and achieve our vision by following our core beliefs and values.

Our Beliefs

- We believe our clients come first.
- We believe our employees are our greatest asset.
- We believe building relationships and working together are critical to our success as a community of compassionate caregivers.
- We believe we must demonstrate honesty and integrity at all times.
- We believe in providing community service where we live and work.
- We believe it is our responsibility to strengthen the organization's financial foundation and to support its growth.

Our Values

Our work is guided by our fundamental values of compassion, excellence, and reliability.

Compassion

Key result: Our clients and their families feel cared for and supported.

Key actions:

- Work with a spirit of universal faith, hope, and love.
- Demonstrate exceptional care and kindness to others. Be led by our hearts.
- Be respectful. Treat others the way they wish to be treated.
- Listen closely, show empathy, and respond to the needs of others.
- Be friendly. Let our smiles be seen and felt.

Excellence

Key result: We provide home health care to our clients with the highest professional, ethical, and safety standards.

Key actions:

- Consistently demonstrate the highest level of skill, competence, and sound judgment in our work.
- Demonstrate honesty, commitment, and loyalty to our clients and their families, to fellow employees, and to our organization.
- Strive to provide the very best service to our clients. Set specific goals and work hard and efficiently to achieve them.
- Continuously improve our work through evaluation, education, and training.
- Recognize and reward those who set and maintain the highest standards of excellence.

Reliability

Key result: Our clients and their families can rely on us and are able to live their lives to the fullest, with a sense of well-being, dignity, and trust.

Key actions:

- Keep our commitments as promised.
- Consistently deliver expected services.
- Fulfill our clients' needs promptly and thoroughly.
- Be creative, flexible, and determined—get the job done for our clients.
- Communicate clearly and consistently with clients and fellow employees.

Index

Page numbers in **boldface** indicate illustrations and captions.